Journey To Wellness Cookbook

100 easy plant-based recipes
with traditional and Thermomix cooking methods

Sacha Hooper

Published by Sacha Hooper

Copywrite © 2022. All rights reserved. No portion of this publication may be used, reproduced or transmitted by any means, digital, electronic, mechanical, photocopy or recording without written permission of the publisher, except in the case of brief quotations within critical articles or reviews.

Photography – Back cover and all recipe photography by Sacha Hooper. Front cover and category section images by Lanie Sims Photography.

ISBN: 978-0-6455980-0-1 (paperback)
First edition, 2022

For book orders and enquiries, contact:

Sacha Hooper

detoxifyandnourish@gmail.com

www.detoxifyandnourish.com.au

Instagram: @detoxify_and_nourish

Facebook: Detoxify and Nourish

MY JOURNEY TO WELLNESS

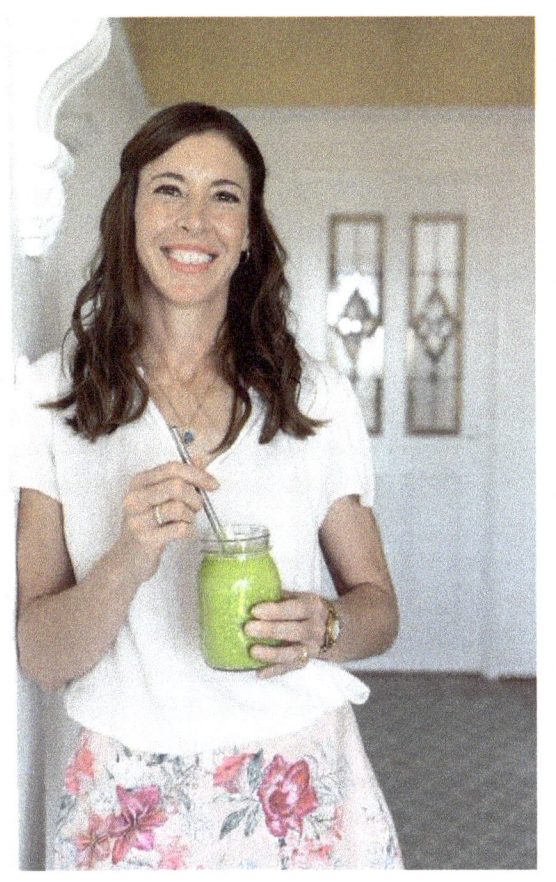

I am so honoured you have been drawn to this book. I know it will inspire you to create easy nourishing healthy meals for you and your family. I truly believe the plants on our beautiful earth give us amazing nourishment and have the ability to heal our bodies.

My journey to wellness began from dealing with my own health issues, which culminated in me growing a large cyst on my thyroid and a specialist telling me that without immediate surgery, I could have as little as 1 week left to live! After the surgery I was told that I would need to take thyroid and anxiety medication for the rest of my life, which I didn't like the sound of, so I decided to take my health into my own hands. I began reading labels on food packets, I eliminated toxic additives, changed the products my family used on our bodies and within our home and I began looking for more natural holistic options. Then we changed our diet as we moved into a plant-based way of eating, and this is when we noticed the biggest improvement in our health.

Not only has my own health with my thyroid issues, menstrual issues, anxiety issues, skin issues and general wellbeing all greatly improved, but my husband who joined me on this journey has lost weight, feels more energised, is less bloated and his emotions are more balanced. His chronic sinus and heartburn issues have disappeared too. By removing animal products from our family diet, beginning with the elimination of dairy, our son's severe Asthma reduced dramatically. We were no longer regular visitors to the emergency ward at the hospital or respiratory specialist clinics. Over time, he was no longer triggered by grasses, viral infections, or a change in the weather. His years of suffering with life threating symptoms ended and he became a happy little boy who had energy! Our daughters' constant ear, nose and throat infections also disappeared. Our bodies found harmony and balance.

So, with a full heart, I dedicate this book to my beautiful family. To my husband Brad, thank you for always supporting and encouraging me on every step of our life journey together. Even when I first suggested cutting out meat and dairy – you embraced the challenge and have never looked back as the health benefits were so clear to see. To my daughter Rhianna, thank you for always making me laugh during my food flops, for helping me challenge myself and encouraging me to keep following my dream. To my son Ryan, thank you for always being willing to try the food I create and for giving me a big smile and a 'thumbs up'. I love you all and I am so happy our collective health has improved so much as we continue our journey to detoxify and nourish.

Sacha xx

This book has been created from my deep passion for holistic health
and having personally experienced the benefits from embracing a plant-based lifestyle.

The body has an amazing ability to regain and maintain wellness when we
detoxify from meat, dairy and all the additives often found in processed foods
and nourish it with wholesome, fresh, natural ingredients straight from mother earth.

These recipes have come into this world via me turning some old family favourites
that have been passed down through the generations into plant-based versions,
and from having fun in my kitchen creating some tasty new food.

It is filled with simple family friendly recipes that have taken years of
creating and tweaking so that our kids enjoyed them just as much as us.

You won't find any fancy ingredients,
in fact, you probably have most of the ingredients you need
in your pantry right now!

I am so excited to share all these recipes with you.
I hope you enjoy them as much as we do and find the incredible
health benefits of eating plant-based.

I hope this book helps to inspire and empower you on your
own 'journey to wellness'.

COOKING METHODS

There are 2 ways of cooking for almost every recipe within this book. All 100 recipes have a Traditional method of cooking, while 88 also have a corresponding Thermomix (TM) method. This is because sometimes the recipe just requires a traditional approach or the use of another appliance like a juicer, which will produce a better result.

For those that find the chopping, mixing and stirring therapeutic - you can follow the Traditional method.

For those wanting the support of an appliance to measure, blend and cook - the Thermomix method will allow you to do this so that you can get on with other aspects of family life. In some Thermomix recipes, I have cut vegetables by hand to keep their shape, or cooked the quinoa / rice separately in a saucepan to reduce the overall cooking time. I have included 'how to cook quinoa / rice in the Thermomix' instructions below.

I have created these recipes using the TM5. However, these can also be used in the TM6 and TM31. Please note, the TM31 bowl capacity is a little smaller then the TM5, so just be mindful to not go over the max line when cooking recipes with a lot of ingredients or liquid.

HOW TO COOK QUINOA / RICE IN THE THERMOMIX IN 6 EASY STEPS

1. Rinse the quinoa or rice under water first. The amount doesn't matter, you can do 50g - 200g.
2. Add it to the TM simmering basket.
3. Insert the simmering basket into the TM.
4. Add 1000g filtered water.
5. Cook for 15 MIN / 100°C / SP 4.
6. Discard the liquid once cooked.

A GUIDED SHOPPING LIST

Provided over the following pages are the main ingredients that I use in these recipes. I have also included a brief explanation of the key health benefits these ingredients have to offer. Having these ingredients in your kitchen will allow you to easily prepare each of the recipes in this cookbook.

- **Oats** — Are loaded with fibre and minerals and have beneficial effects on the gastrointestinal tract. Try to buy organic where possible to avoid pesticides.

- **Chia Seeds** — Contain fibre, calcium, iron and omega-3. They improve digestive health and provide sustainable energy.

- **Flax Seeds** — Are full of Omega-3 and protein. They are great for heart health. Ground flax seeds mixed with a little water makes an excellent egg substitute.

- **Almonds** — A handful of almonds can reduce hunger, assist with blood sugar control and lower cholesterol. They are full of antioxidants.

- **Cashew Nuts** — Are rich in protein, magnesium, zinc and iron. These help the body to function well. When cashews are soaked and blended, they make excellent dairy alternatives, for products like plant based sour cream, milk and cheese.

- **Macadamia Nuts** — Help reduce inflammation and are rich in heart healthy monounsaturated fats.

- **Walnuts** — Are great for brain health. They even look like little brains!

- **Organic Cacao Powder** — Is chocolate in its purest form. It is packed with antioxidants, vitamins, minerals and magnesium. It is also dairy and gluten free.

- **Maca Powder** — Boosts energy, improves mood, helps with fertility, balances hormones and eases menopausal symptoms. Make sure to buy a good quality organic brand.

- **Organic Coconut Oil** — Has many anti-inflammatory benefits. Organic virgin coconut oil is a pure cold pressed product.

- **Olive Oil** — Extra virgin olive oil (EVOO) is incredibly healthy due to its high level of antioxidants, which can benefit your heart, brain and joints.

- **Wholemeal Flour** — Is packed with nutrients, vitamins and fibre as it hasn't been refined or bleached, unlike white flour.

- **Organic Shredded Coconut** — I only buy organic, as Sulphites (200 numbers) are found in non-organic shredded coconut and are linked with asthma. Inflammation from sulphites may present itself as mild respiratory symptoms, wheezing or be potentially life threatening.

- **Pure Maple Syrup** — Contains antioxidants, magnesium, zinc, calcium and potassium. It also has antimicrobial properties, helping your body to fight harmful bacteria.

- **Rice Malt Syrup** — Is a sweetener made from brown rice and is an alternative to honey.

- **Nut Butter** — Is full of heart healthy fats, protein and fibre. It is easy to make your own nut butter and I have included a recipe in this book for you to try.

- Organic Tamari Sauce — Is an alternative to soy sauce, containing less salt. Organic tamari sauce is made using organic, non-GMO soybeans which is beneficial to your health.

- Tinned Tomatoes — Tomatoes are full of antioxidants, potassium, vitamins B and E and help to protect your cells from any damage.

- Organic Coconut Cream — Contains healthy fats which decrease appetite and increase energy. It is a great alternative to dairy full cream products. It is also high in potassium which is critical for maintaining the health of every cell in your body.

- Tinned Lentils — Are high in protein and fibre and are a great substitute for meat. They are full of potassium, folate and iron.

- Tinned Black Beans — Contain antioxidants, protein, fibre and are filled with phytochemicals that help to protect your cells and heart.

- Tinned Kidney Beans — Are a complete protein and interestingly are great for your kidneys (being kidney shaped and all). Like other beans, they contain fibre, protein, antioxidants and flavonoids – shown to provide defence against cancer.

- Tinned Jackfruit — A superfood containing antioxidants, vitamins B6, B1, C, A, calcium, potassium, iron, magnesium, fibre and omega-3 which is amazing for your immune system.

- Pasta — Is made from grains and is a great source of fibre and energy. Grains are often sprayed with pesticides though, so try to buy organic wherever possible as consuming pesticides can cause an irritable bowel over a period of time.

- Rice — Rice that has the bran layer intact, (e.g. brown rice, red rice, black rice) has more nutritional value than white rice. It is full of antioxidants and has a lower GI which is great for diabetics.

- Dried Herbs and Spices — Generally, dried herbs are stronger than fresh herbs. You only need a small amount too. Herbs have been used for centuries for their culinary and medicinal properties.

- Plant-based Milk — This includes milk made from nuts like almonds, cashews and macadamias, or oats, soy, rice, sesame and coconut. Plant-based milk is full of nutrients that we can digest easily, unlike cow milk which can be very inflammatory to the human body, often irritating the airways / respiratory system.

- Medjool Dates — Have plant compounds that can reduce inflammation, stimulate the immune system, prevent DNA damage and improve and regulate hormones.

- Bananas — Contain a protein that's converted into serotonin once digested. This makes you feel happy and smile. The banana is even the shape of a smile.

- Avocado — They are shaped like the cervix and are excellent for womb health.

- Berries — Are a superfood! They are some of the best foods you can have to boost your immune system. Berries can also be in the top 10 dirty dozen as they have soft skin which pesticides and chemicals can easily penetrate. Soak your berries with 1 cup apple cider vinegar in a sink of water to help remove pesticides or purchase some organic ones.

- **Citrus Fruits** — Are an excellent source of vitamin C which boosts your immune system. Although citrus is acidic, it turns alkaline in your body which keeps acid in the stomach down and your pH levels balanced. Citrus fruits also help to cleanse the entire lymphatic system.

- **Lemons** — Are full of electrolytes and squeezed into warm water can help to detox the body.

- **Apples** — Are excellent for cleaning the lymphatic system. Keeping your lymph clear of toxic buildup improves your immunity and health. Eat them fresh or juiced.

- **Mushrooms** — Are full of iron and are beneficial for a healthy functioning thyroid. They also contain vitamin D. By placing 3 mushrooms in the sun for 1 hour (gills up), the vitamin D content increases, which is beneficial for our daily levels. Shiitake mushrooms are best, but button mushrooms work too.

- **Pineapple** — Supports and detoxes the thyroid. They are full of vitamins and minerals which helps to aid digestion and increase immune system strength.

- **Leafy Greens** — Are known for their cancer fighting compounds and high iron levels.

- **Broccoli** — The #1 vegetable in fighting cancer cells. Broccoli also looks like the bronchi and is known to have compounds that clean harmful bacteria from the lungs.

- **Cauliflower** — Is a cruciferous vegetable like the broccoli. It is full of anti-inflammatory, anti-viral and anti-bacterial properties.

- **Carrots** — Are full of nutrients to protect eye health. Interestingly, when cut into circles they look just like an eye.

- **Celery** — Is full of calcium and helps to keep your bones strong.

- **Potatoes** — Contain fibre which is great for digestive health.

- **Sweet Potato** — Helps to balance the endocrine system. This is great for women experiencing menopause and hot flashes. Sweet Potatoes are good for pancreatic health too.

- **Eggplant** — Is very nourishing for the gall bladder.

- **Onion** — Has digestive benefits and helps to maintain levels of good bacteria. They are also rich in vitamin C which helps to boost your immunity.

- **Garlic** — Has been used for centuries to ward off coughs and colds.

- **Tomatoes** — Tomatoes have 4 chambers just like our heart and are great for heart health.

- **Pumpkin** — Is one of the greatest sources of vitamin A. They are also rich in antioxidants to keep your skin, eyes, immune system and blood pressure healthy.

- **Organic Tofu** — Contains plant estrogen which is great for reducing hot flashes in women. Organic is important, as soy crops are often sprayed heavily with chemicals.

- **Fresh Herbs** — Add flavour and can help protect the body with their health boosting compounds.

THE RECIPE COLLECTION

BREAKFAST — **12**
- Avocado Smash — 13
- Beans on Toast — 14
- Fluffy Pancakes — 15
- Berry Tasty Pancakes — 16
- Easy Cereal — 17
- Nutty Muesli — 18
- Coco Puffs — 19
- Chia Seed Pudding — 20
- Cacao Granola — 21
- Breakfast Cookie — 22

DRINKS — **23**
- Cleansing Green Juice — 24
- Immune Boost Juice — 25
- Tropical Juice — 26
- Chocolate Protein Shake — 27
- Nutty Smoothie — 28
- Green Goodness Smoothie — 29
- Berry Bliss Smoothie — 30
- Cashew Nut Milk — 31
- Almond Milk — 32
- Mulled Apple Juice — 33
- Spiced Hot Chocolate — 34
- Turmeric Tea — 35

SNACKS — **36**
- Raw Peanut Butter Cookies — 37
- Macadamia Choc Cookies — 38
- Cashew Sesame Slice — 39
- Fruit Nut Slice — 40
- Hazelnut Protein Balls — 41
- Banana Cinnamon Bread — 42
- Anzac Slice — 43
- Crispy Peanut Butter Bars — 44
- Salted Caramel Raw Balls — 45
- No Bake Oat Bars — 46
- Peppermint Protein Balls — 47
- Nut Free Bliss Balls — 48
- The Big Cookie — 49

Peanut Butter Bliss Balls	50
Lime Bliss Balls	51
Raw Fudgy Brownie	52
Muesli Bars	53
Choc Chip Bliss Balls (and Cookies)	54
Raw Orange Almond Slice	55
Carrot Walnut Bread	56
Nourish Slice	57
Mud Muffins	58
Sweet n Salty Nuts	59
Kale Chips	60
CONDIMENTS	**61**
Cashnew Nut Butter	62
Raspberry Chia Jam	63
Cashew Parmesan	64
Vegetable Stock Paste	65
Cashew Sour Cream	66
Cashew Aioli	67
Creamy Dill Dressing	68
Mexican Spice Mix	69
Tuscan Seasoning Mix	70
Chocolate Drinking Powder	71
Chocolate Dipping Sauce	72
DINNERS	**73**
Creamy Tomato Pasta	74
Stuffed Mushrooms	75
Vegetable Pie	76
Quinoa Bolognese	77
Curried Coconut Pumpkin Soup	78
Cheesy Broccoli Pasta	79
Jackfruit Tacos	80
Zucchini Cauliflower Corn Soup	81
Tuscan Quinoa Balls	82
Minestrone Soup	84
Basil Pesto Pasta	85
Nourish Stew	86
Roast Pumpkin Risotto	87
Falafels	89
Oven Vegetable Bake	90
Stir Fry Asian Noodles	91
Nachos	92
Hearty Noodle Soup	93

Vegetable Laksa	94
Spiced Vege Soup	95
Chickpea Corn Bowl	96
Maple Roasted Couscous Salad	97
Vege Enchiladas	98
Sweet n Sour Crispy Tofu	100
Coriander Lime Cauli Rice	101
Burger Patties	102
Eggplant Parmigana	103
Green Curry	104
Cauliflower Bites	105
Seasoned Wedges	106
Sweet Potato Pie	107
Mexican Burrito Bowl	109
Lentil Lasagne	110
Miso Soup	112
DESSERT	**113**
Chocolate Mint Mousse	114
Berry Sorbet	115
Peanut Butter Chocolate	116
Easy Raw Chocolate	117
Apple Crumble	118
Salted Caramel Ice Cream	119
Chewy Choc Caramel Fudge	120
Peppermint Ice	121
Fudge Choc Pops	122

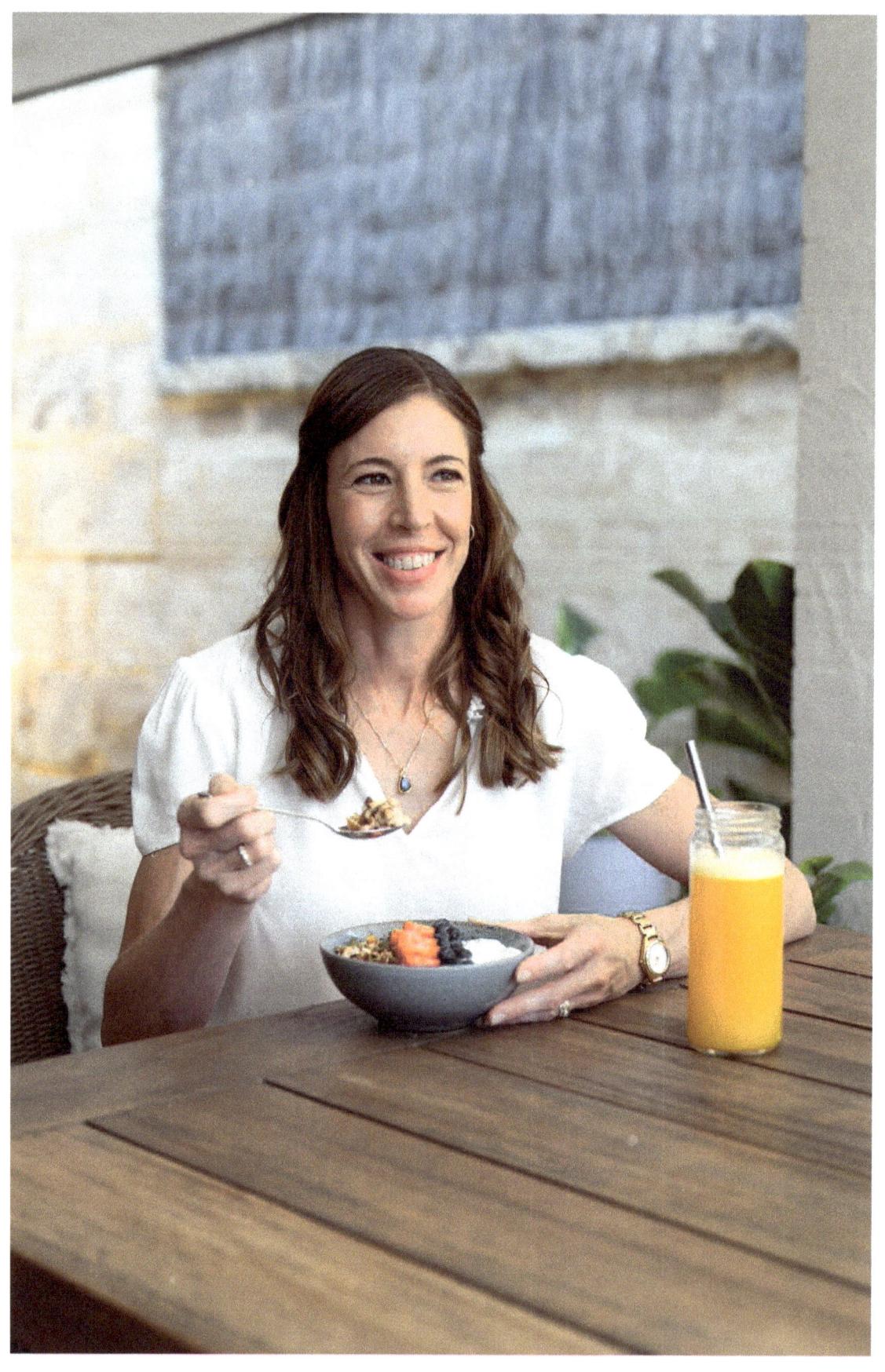

BREAKFAST

BREAKFAST

AVOCADO SMASH

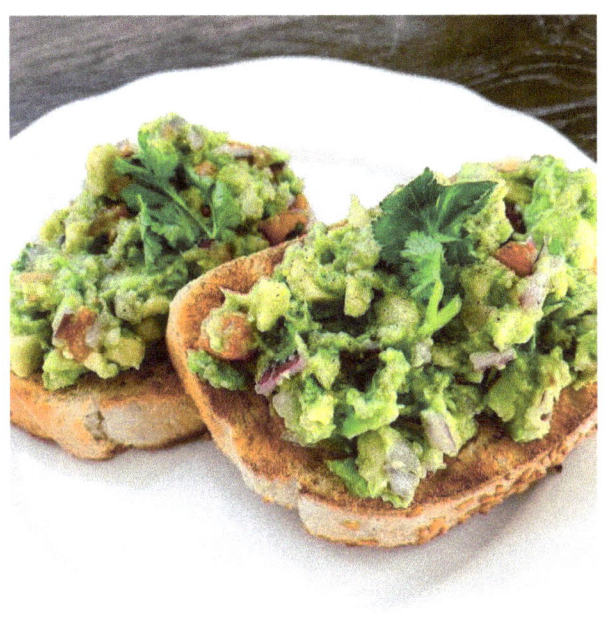

Prep. Time:	Make Time:	Serves:
5 min	1 min	2-4

DIRECTIONS – Traditional Only

Traditional ~ Slice the avocados in half and remove the seeds. Scoop out the avocado flesh into a bowl and mash with a fork and set aside.

Finely dice the tomato, onion and coriander. Add these plus the lemon juice to the bowl and stir together.

Toast up some fresh bread and serve the avocado smash on top.

NOTES

Garnish with fresh coriander leaves.

INGREDIENTS

- 2 Ripe Avocados
- ½ Roma Tomato
- ¼ Red Onion
- 2 Tbsp Fresh Coriander + some leaves for garnish
- ¼ Lemon (juice only)

BREAKFAST

BEANS ON TOAST

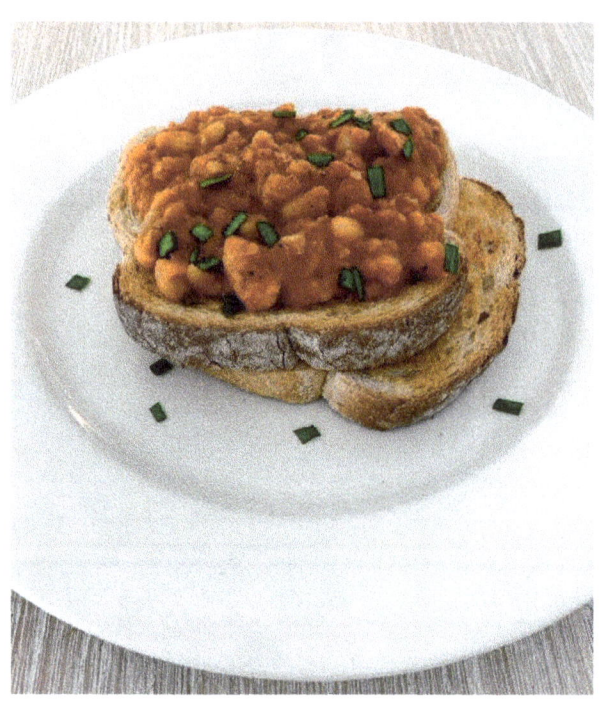

Prep. Time:	Cook Time:	Serves:
5 min	7 min	3-4

DIRECTIONS

Traditional ~ Peel and finely dice the garlic and onion. Add these to a saucepan with the olive oil and sauté for 2 MIN.

Rinse and drain the cannellini beans. Add these plus all remaining ingredients and stir together for 5 MIN over a low heat.

Thermomix ~ Place the peeled garlic and onion into the TM bowl and chop for 1 SEC / SP 7. Scrape down the sides of the bowl. Add the olive oil and sauté for 3 MIN / VAROMA / SP 1.

Rinse and drain the cannellini beans. Add these plus all remaining ingredients. Cook for 5 MIN / 70°C / REVERSE / SP 2.

~ ~ ~ ~ ~ ~ ~ ~ ~ ~ ~ ~ ~ ~ ~

Toast up some fresh bread and serve the beans on top.

NOTES

Garnish with fresh herbs if desired. This recipe makes enough beans for 6 pieces of toast.

INGREDIENTS

- 2 Garlic Cloves
- 75g (½) Brown Onion
- 15g (1 Tbsp) Olive Oil
- 180g (¾ cup) Passata Sauce
- 20g (1 Tbsp) Tomato Paste
- 60g (¼ cup) Filtered Water
- ½ tsp ground Paprika
- ¼ tsp ground Cumin
- ¼ tsp dried Basil
- ¼ tsp Fine Sea Salt
- ¼ tsp Fine Black Pepper
- ¼ tsp Raw Sugar
- 1 x 400g tinned Cannellini Beans
- Garlic Chives (for garnish)

BREAKFAST

FLUFFY PANCAKES

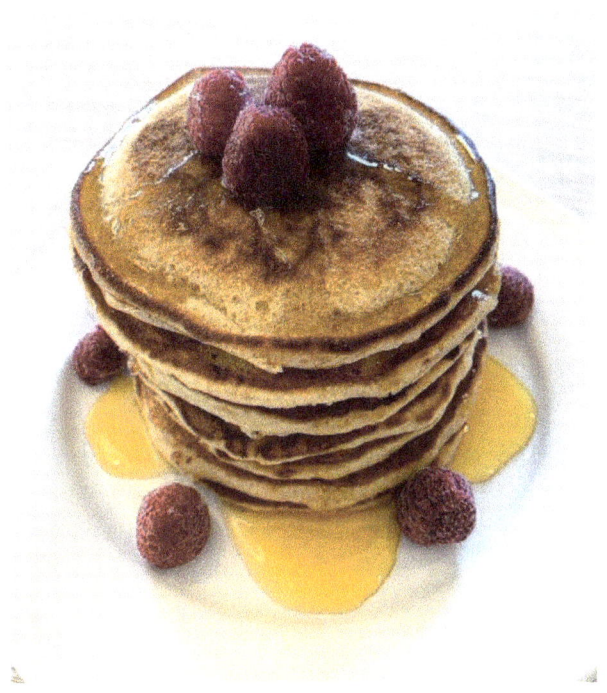

INGREDIENTS

- 180g (¾ cup) Plant-based Milk
- 15g (1 Tbsp) Apple Cider Vinegar
- 120g (¾ cup) Wholemeal Plain Flour
- ½ tsp Baking Powder
- ½ tsp Bi-Carb Soda
- Pinch of fine Sea Salt
- 40g (2 Tbsp) Maple Syrup
- 5g (1 tsp) Organic Vanilla Bean Paste
- 90g (½ cup) Chocolate Chips (optional)

TOPPINGS
- Pure Maple Syrup
- Organic Raspberries
- Hemp Seeds

Prep. Time: 10 min Cook Time: 10 min Serves: 3-4

DIRECTIONS

Traditional ~ In a small bowl combine the milk and apple cider vinegar. Stir together and allow to stand for 5 MIN.

Add all the remaining ingredients into a medium sized bowl. Stir together. Then pour in the milk and cider mixture and stir until combined. Fold in the chocolate chips if desired.

~ ~ ~ ~ ~ ~ ~ ~ ~ ~ ~ ~ ~ ~ ~

Thermomix ~ In a small bowl combine the milk and apple cider vinegar. Stir together and allow to stand for 5 MIN.

To the TM bowl, add the remaining ingredients. Then pour in the milk and cider mixture. Mix for 10 SEC / SP 4. Scrape down the sides of the bowl and stir again for 10 SEC / SP 4. If desired, add in the chocolate chips and stir for
6 SEC / REVERSE / SP 4.

~ ~ ~ ~ ~ ~ ~ ~ ~ ~ ~ ~ ~ ~ ~

Lightly oil a large frypan, and over a medium heat, pour in small amounts of the mixture. When it begins to bubble, flip the pancakes over carefully and cook the other side until brown. Repeat this for the remainder of the pancake mixture.

NOTES

Top your pancake stack with maple syrup, raspberries and hemp seeds.

BREAKFAST

BERRY TASTY PANCAKES

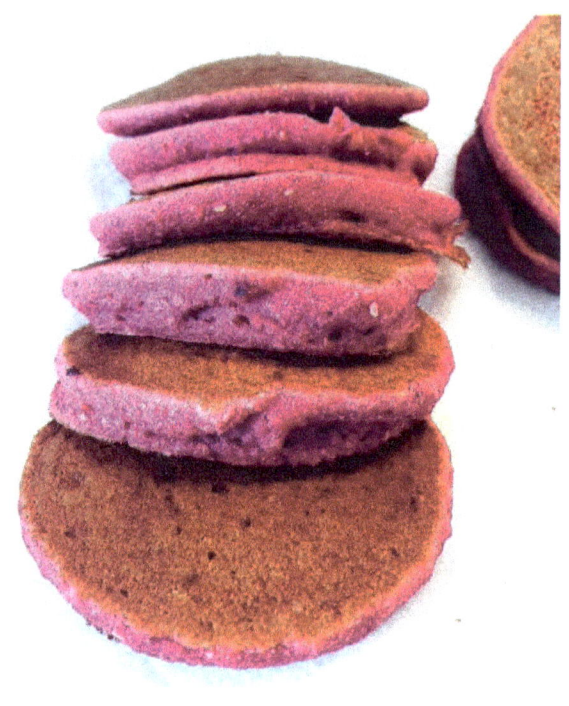

Prep. Time:	Cook Time:	Serves:
10 min	10 min	4

DIRECTIONS

1. Prepare the flax egg by combining 1 Tbsp of flax meal (ground flax seeds) with 2 ½ Tbsp filtered water. Allow this to sit for 5 minutes to thicken.

Traditional ~ Add the raspberries and the cored and quartered apple to a food processor. Blitz together. Scrape down the sides of the bowl. Add all remaining ingredients, including the flax egg and mix to combine.

Thermomix ~ Add the raspberries and the cored and quartered apple into the TM bowl and blitz for 4 SEC / SP 9. Scrape down the sides of the bowl. Add the remaining ingredients, including the flax egg and mix for 20 SEC / SP 5.

~ ~ ~ ~ ~ ~ ~ ~ ~ ~ ~ ~ ~ ~ ~

Lightly oil a large frypan, and over a medium heat, pour in small amounts of the mixture. Flip the pancakes over once browned. Repeat until all the batter is gone.

INGREDIENTS

- 1 Flax Egg
- 110g (1 cup) Organic Frozen Raspberries
- 200g (2 small) Red Apples – core removed
- 200g (1 ¼ cups) Wholemeal Plain Flour
- 10g (2 tsp) Baking Powder
- 5g (1 tsp) Organic Vanilla Bean Paste
- 30g (2 Tbsp) Raw Sugar
- 250g (1 cup) Almond Milk
- 5g (1 tsp) Organic Beetroot Powder

NOTES

Serve with your favourite toppings.

BREAKFAST

EASY CEREAL

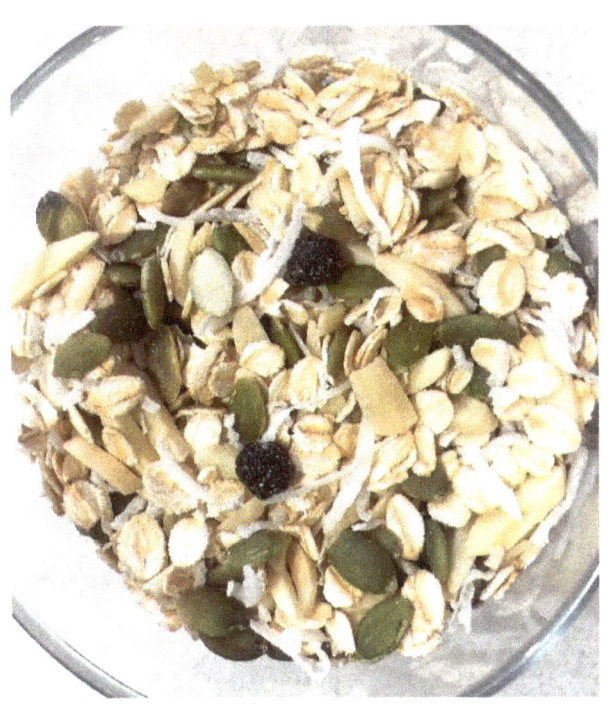

Prep. Time:	Cook Time:	Makes:
5 min	20 min	630g

DIRECTIONS

Traditional ~ Combine all the ingredients into a large bowl and stir to combine.

Thermomix ~ Combine all the ingredients into the TM bowl and mix for 10 SEC / REVERSE / SP 1.

~~~~~~~~~~~~~~~~

Line a baking tray with baking paper and empty the cereal mix onto it.

Bake in the oven at 150°C for 20 MIN to lightly toast the cereal.

INGREDIENTS

- 220g (2 cups) Organic Rolled Oats
- 160g (1 cup) Pepita Seeds
- 110g (1 cup) Slivered Almonds
- 100g (1 cup) Organic Shredded Coconut
- 25g (¼ cup) Organic Dried Blueberries / Goji Berries / Dried Cranberries

NOTES

Store in an airtight container for up to 4 weeks.

BREAKFAST

NUTTY MUESLI

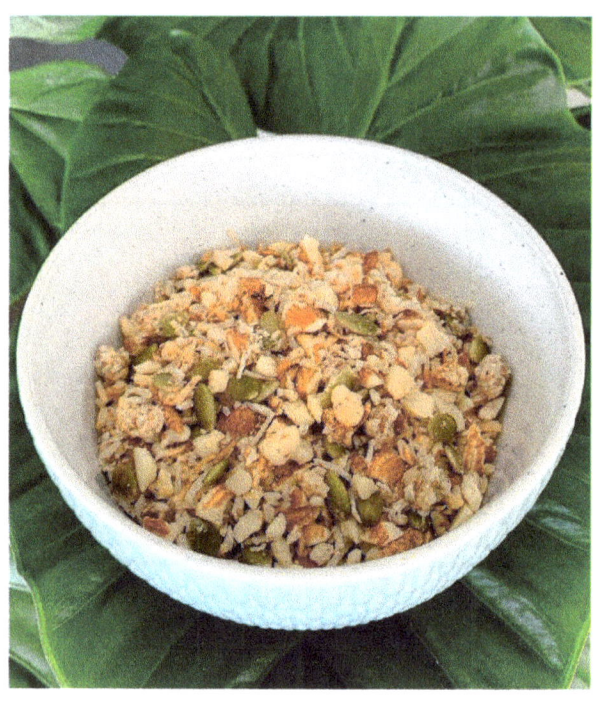

Prep. Time:	Cook Time:	Makes:
5 min	12 min	520g

DIRECTIONS

Traditional ~ Place the almonds, macadamia and brazil nuts into a food processor and blitz it up (the mixture should be mostly fine with some chunkier bits). Tip this into a large bowl. Add the remaining ingredients and mix until combined.

Thermomix ~ Place the almonds, macadamia and brazil nuts into the TM bowl and chop for 3 SEC / SP 6. Add the remaining ingredients and mix for 15 SEC / REVERSE / SP 3.

~ ~ ~ ~ ~ ~ ~ ~ ~ ~ ~ ~ ~ ~ ~

Line a baking tray with baking paper and spread the muesli evenly onto the tray. Bake in the oven at 180°C for 12 MIN, stirring halfway.

Once cooked, remove the tray from the oven and allow it to cool completely – it will get crunchier as it cools down.

INGREDIENTS

- 225g (1 ½ cups) Natural Almonds
- 50g (⅓ cup) Macadamia Nuts
- 50g (⅓ cup) Brazil Nuts
- 50g (⅓ cup) Pepita Seeds
- 70g (1 cup) Organic Shredded Coconut
- 5g (1 tsp) Chia Seeds
- 5g (1 tsp) Organic Vanilla Bean Paste
- 40g (2 Tbsp) Organic Rice Malt Syrup
- 15g (1 Tbsp) Organic Coconut Oil

NOTES

Store in an airtight container for up to 4 weeks.

Serve with your choice of plant-based milk, fresh fruit and a sprinkle of cinnamon if desired.

BREAKFAST

COCO PUFFS

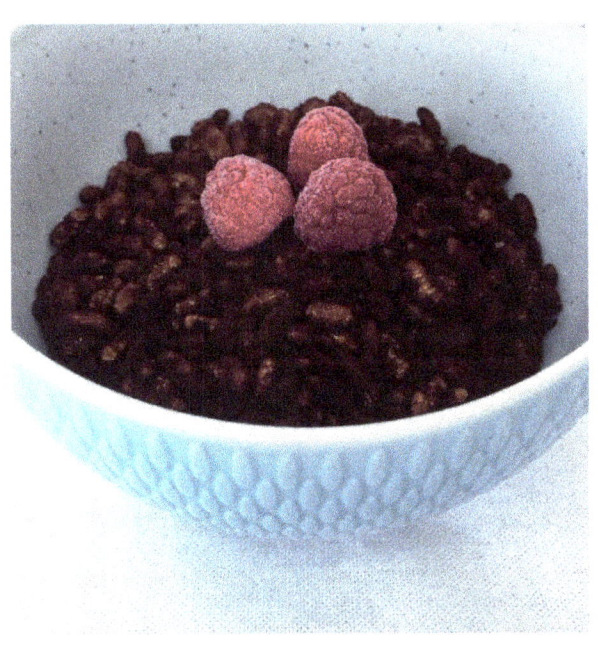

INGREDIENTS

- 140g (4 cups) Puffed Rice (Rice Bubbles)
- 80g (⅓ cup) Organic Coconut Oil
- 110g (⅓ cup) Pure Maple Syrup
- 20g (4 Tbsp) Organic Cacao Powder

Prep. Time:	Cook Time:	Makes:
5 min	30 min	330g

DIRECTIONS

Traditional ~ Melt the coconut oil, then pour the liquid into a large bowl. Add the maple syrup and cacao powder and mix to combine. Add the rice bubbles and mix until evenly coated.

Thermomix ~ Add the coconut oil and melt for 2 MIN / 60°C / SP 1. Add the maple syrup and cacao powder and mix for 10 SEC / SP 4. Add the rice bubbles and stir for 30 SEC / REVERSE / SP 1.

~ ~ ~ ~ ~ ~ ~ ~ ~ ~ ~ ~ ~ ~ ~

Line a baking tray with baking paper. Spread the mixture evenly onto the tray. Bake in the oven at 120°C for 30 MIN, stirring every 10 MIN.

Allow to cool completely on the tray before serving.

NOTES

Store in an airtight container for up to 1 week.

Serve with your choice of plant-based milk and fresh fruit if desired.

BREAKFAST

CHIA SEED PUDDING

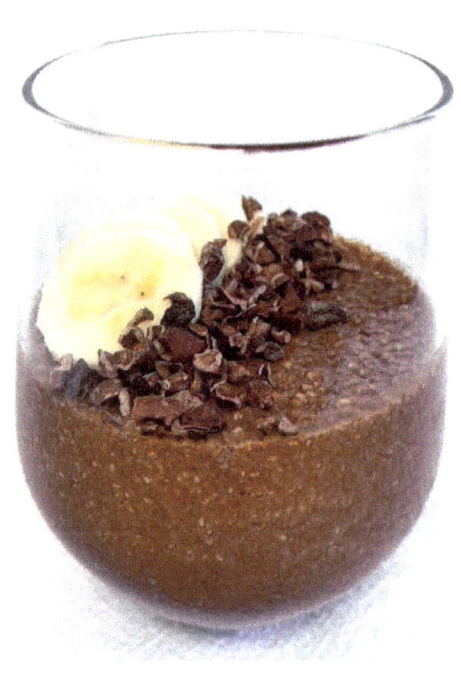

INGREDIENTS

- 90g (½ cup) Chia Seeds
- 380g (1 ½ cups) Organic Soy Milk
- 80g (4 Tbsp) Pure Maple Syrup
- 10g (2 tsp) Organic Vanilla Bean Paste
- 20g (3 Tbsp) Organic Cacao Powder
- Pinch of Sea Salt

Prep. Time:	Cook Time:	Serves:
5 min	N/A	2

DIRECTIONS

Traditional ~ Add all the ingredients into a medium sized bowl and mix thoroughly.

Thermomix ~ Place all the ingredients into the TM bowl and mix for 7 SEC / SP 7.

~ ~ ~ ~ ~ ~ ~ ~ ~ ~ ~ ~ ~ ~ ~

Pour into 2 cups and place into the fridge to set overnight. Top with your favourite fruit and cacao nibs.

NOTES

For a vanilla alternative, leave out the cacao powder and reduce the maple syrup by 1 Tbsp.

If using almond milk, use a ¼ cup less, as generally it is a thinner consistency.

BREAKFAST

CACAO GRANOLA

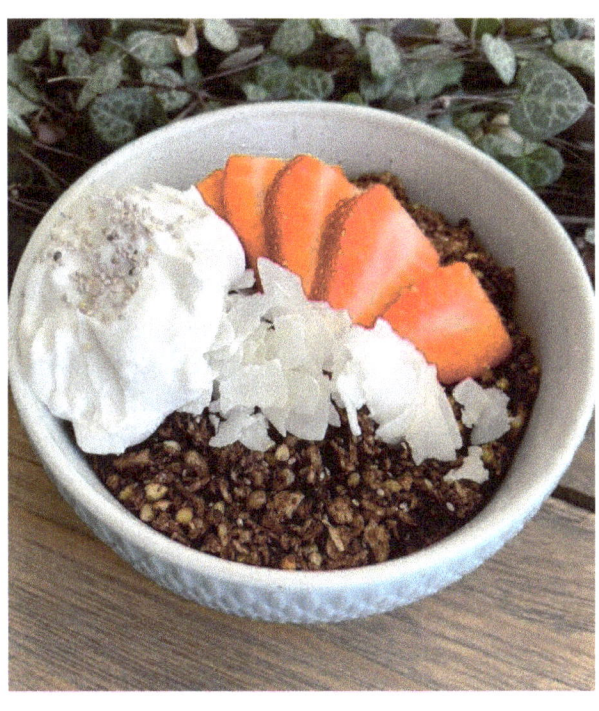

Prep. Time:	Cook Time:	Makes:
5 min	22 min	515g

DIRECTIONS

Traditional ~ Add the oats, buckwheat, chia seeds, cacao powder and salt to a large mixing bowl and stir to combine. Add the vanilla bean paste, maple syrup and cashew nut butter and mix. Fold through the chocolate chips.

Thermomix ~ Add all the ingredients into the TM bowl and mix for 15 SEC / REVERSE / SP 4.

~ ~ ~ ~ ~ ~ ~ ~ ~ ~ ~ ~ ~ ~ ~

Line a baking tray with baking paper. Empty the granola mix onto it, spreading it out evenly. Bake in the oven at 160°C for 22 MIN.

NOTES

Allow the mixture to cool completely before storing it in an airtight container.

Serve with plant-based milk or coconut yoghurt and fresh fruit.

INGREDIENTS

- 250g (2 ¼ cups) Organic Rolled Oats
- 50g (¼ cup) Organic Buckwheat
- 20g (2 Tbsp) Chia Seeds
- 20g (¼ cup) Organic Cacao Powder
- ¼ tsp fine Sea Salt
- 5g (1 tsp) Organic Vanilla Bean Paste
- 120g (¼ cup + 2 Tbsp) Pure Maple Syrup
- 75g (¼ cup) Cashew Nut Butter
- 45g (¼ cup) Chocolate Chips (dairy free)

BREAKFAST

BREAKFAST COOKIE

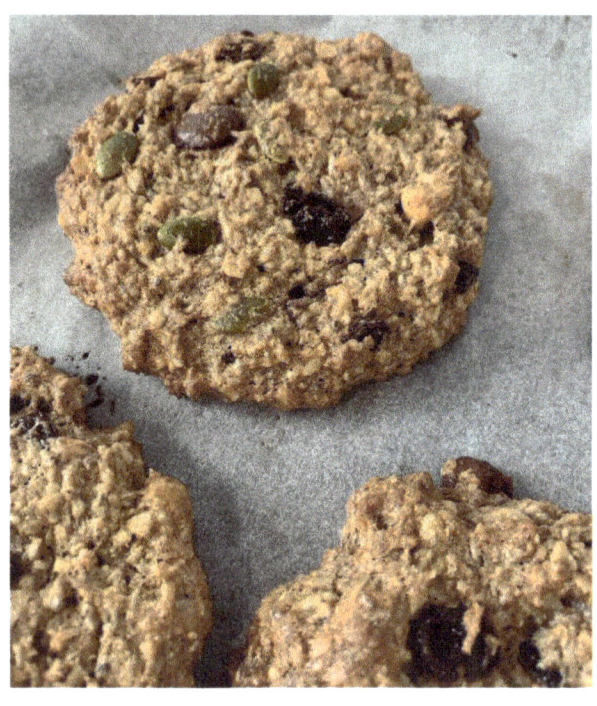

INGREDIENTS

- 100g (1 cup) Organic Rolled Oats
- 50g (½ cup) Almond Meal
- 35g (½ cup) Organic Shredded Coconut
- 5g (1 tsp) Cinnamon Powder
- ½ tsp Baking Powder
- ¼ tsp Fine Sea Salt
- 60g (¼ cup) Organic Coconut Oil (melted)
- 80g (¼ cup) Pure Maple Syrup
- 60g (3 Tbsp) Cashew Nut Butter or PNB*
- 5g (1 tsp) Organic Vanilla Bean Paste
- 40g (¼ cup) Pumpkin Seeds
- 40g (¼ cup) Raisins
- 35g (¼ cup) Macadamia Nut pieces

Prep. Time:	Cook Time:	Makes:
10 min	15 min	6

DIRECTIONS

Traditional ~ In a large bowl, add the oats, almond meal, shredded coconut, cinnamon powder, baking powder and sea salt. Stir together. Add all the remaining ingredients and stir until combined.

Thermomix ~ Add all the ingredients into the TM bowl and mix for 20 SEC / REVERSE / SP 3.

~ ~ ~ ~ ~ ~ ~ ~ ~ ~ ~ ~ ~ ~ ~

Line a baking tray with baking paper. Place 6 large ball shapes of cookie dough onto the tray.

Bake in the oven at 180°C for 18 MIN.

Allow to cool, then store in an airtight container for up to 1 week.

NOTES

To make your own almond meal, simply blitz up ⅓ cup of natural almonds.

*PNB stands for Peanut Butter.

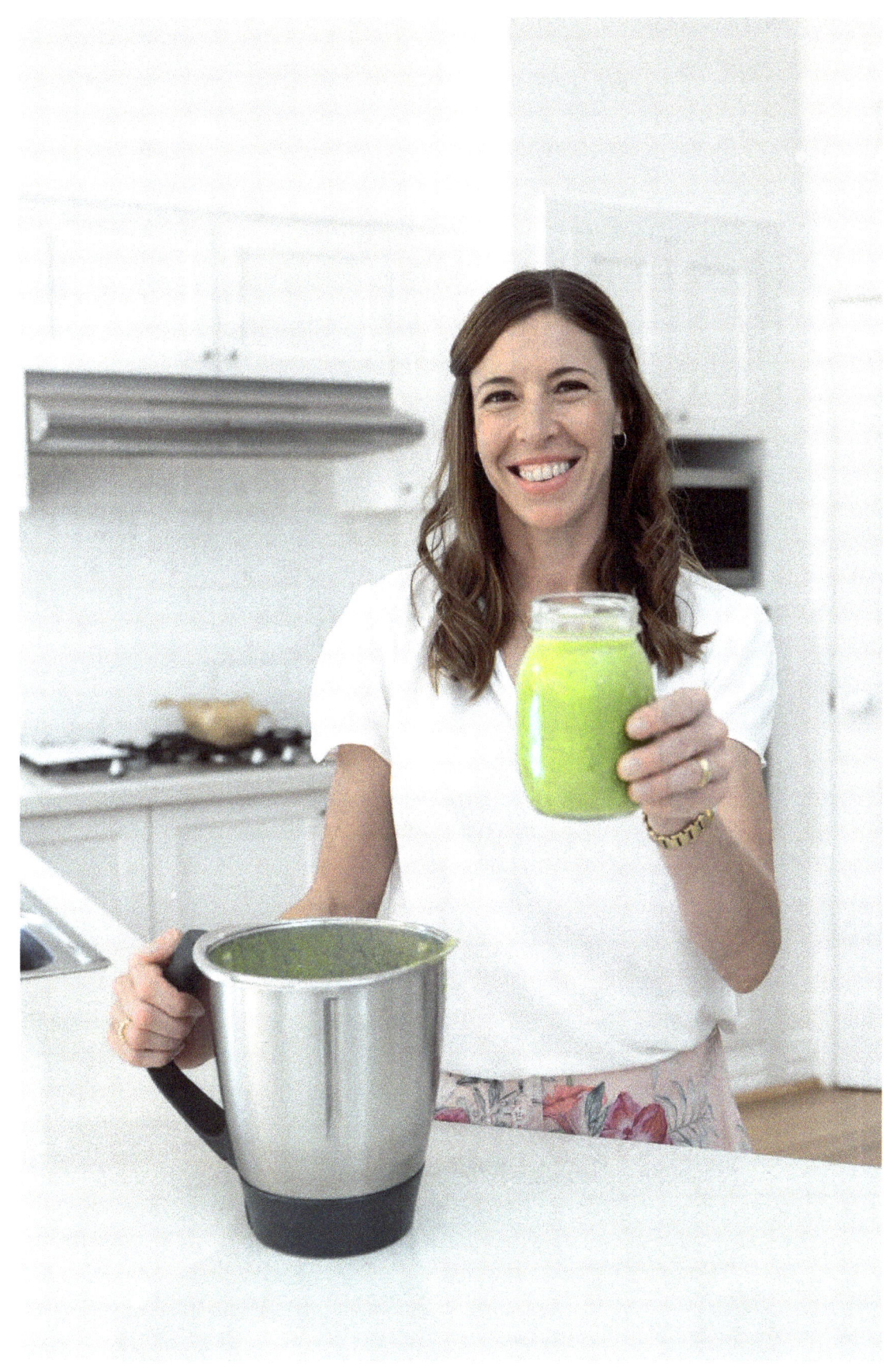

DRINKS

DRINKS

CLEANSING GREEN JUICE

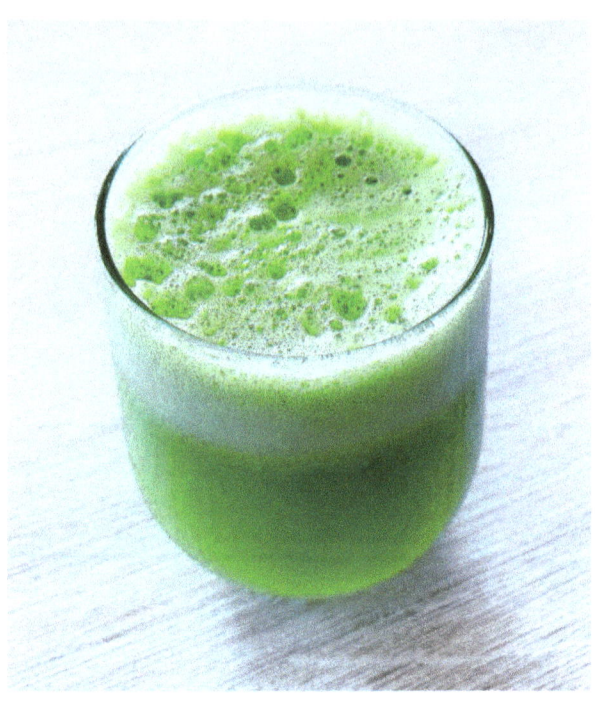

Prep. Time:	Cook Time:	Serves:
5 min	N/A	1-2

DIRECTIONS – Traditional Only

Core the apple. Remove the skin then core and de-seed the pineapple and lemon. Then cut these fruits plus the celery into manageable pieces for the juicer.

Place each ingredient (except the turmeric powder) into a cold pressed juicing machine.

Once your juice is pressed, add the turmeric powder. Stir to combine. Pour into a glass cup and enjoy.

NOTES

This juice is alkaline and is very cleansing for the liver. It's full of antioxidants and is wonderful for the health of the human body.

INGREDIENTS

- 2 Green Apples
- 1 whole Pineapple
- 1 whole Lemon
- 6 sticks of Celery
- 1 Tbsp fresh Coriander
- 2 cm cube fresh Ginger
- ½ tsp ground Turmeric

DRINKS

IMMUNE BOOST JUICE

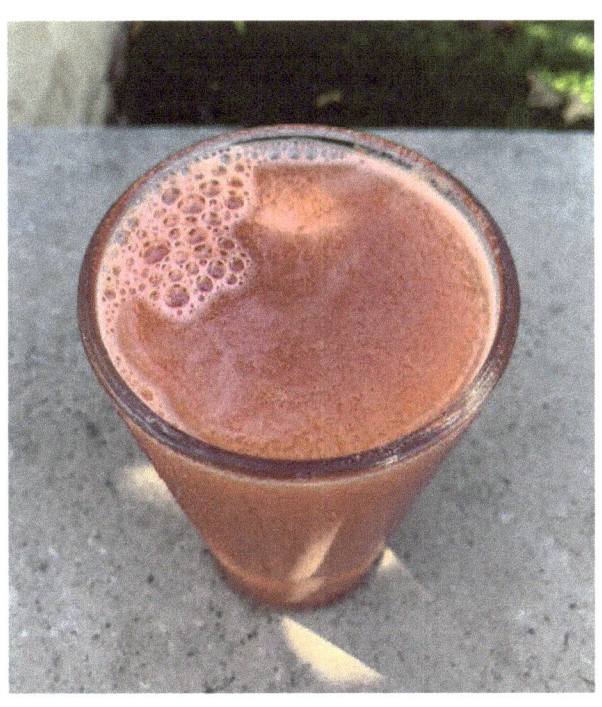

Prep. Time:	Cook Time:	Serves:
10 min	N/A	2

DIRECTIONS – Traditional Only

Peel and remove the skin from all the fruits and vegetables. Cut into manageable pieces for the juicer. Then place each ingredient into a cold pressed juicing machine.

Once your juice is pressed, pour it into a glass cup and enjoy.

NOTES

This juice is immune boosting, high in antioxidants, great for eye vision, heart health and helps to detox the liver.

INGREDIENTS

- 4 medium Carrots
- 4 medium Oranges
- ½ Beetroot
- ½ Dragon Fruit
- 2cm cube Fresh Ginger
- ¼ Lime (juice)

DRINKS

TROPICAL JUICE

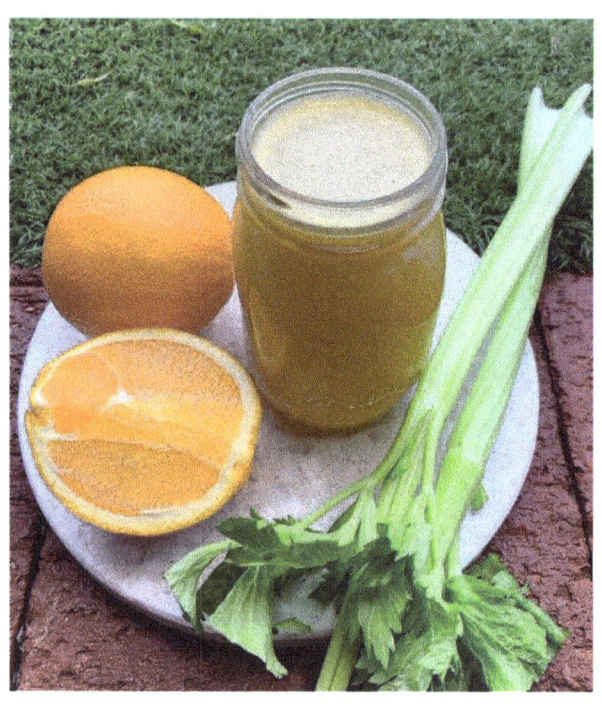

Prep. Time:	Cook Time:	Serves:
10 min	N/A	2

DIRECTIONS – Traditional Only

Remove the skin from pineapple, grapefruit and oranges. Discard the core of the pineapple. Cut all fruits and vegetables into manageable pieces for the juicer.

Place each piece into a cold pressed juicing machine. Once your juice is pressed, pour it into a glass cup and enjoy.

NOTES

This juice is great for thyroid health, bone health and immune health.

INGREDIENTS

- 1 whole Pineapple
- 1 small Grapefruit
- 4 medium Oranges
- 2 sticks Celery

DRINKS

CHOCOLATE PROTEIN SHAKE

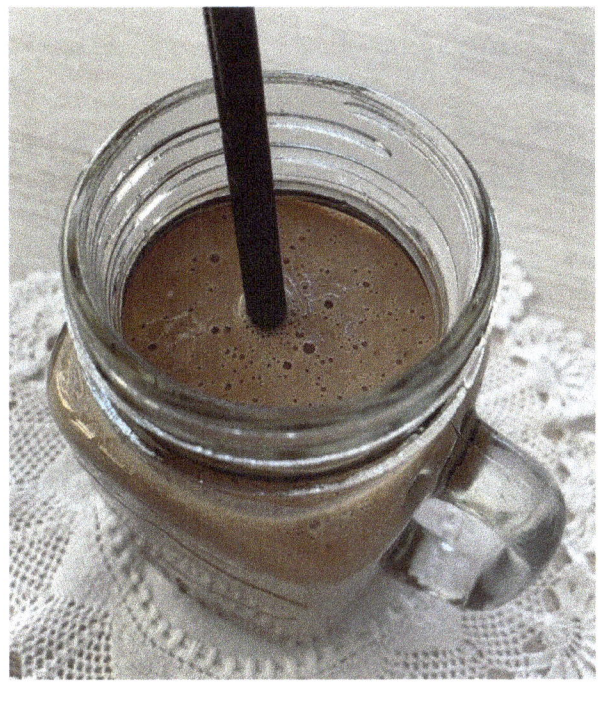

Prep. Time: 5 min

Cook Time: N/A

Serves: 1

DIRECTIONS

Traditional ~ Add all the ingredients into a blender and blend for 1 MIN or until smooth.

Thermomix ~ Add all ingredients into the TM bowl and blitz for 30 SEC / SP 9.

NOTES

This shake is packed full of protein, healthy fats and antioxidants.

INGREDIENTS

- 250g (1 cup) Almond Milk
- 1 frozen Banana
- 1 stick Celery
- Handful Spinach Leaves
- Handful of sliced Zucchini
- 20g (1 Tbsp) Nut Butter
- 5g (1 Tbsp) Organic Cacao Powder
- 1 scoop of Chocolate Plant-based Protein Powder
- 5g (1 tsp) Flax Seeds
- 5g (1 tsp) Maca Powder (optional)

BREAKFAST

NUTTY SMOOTHIE

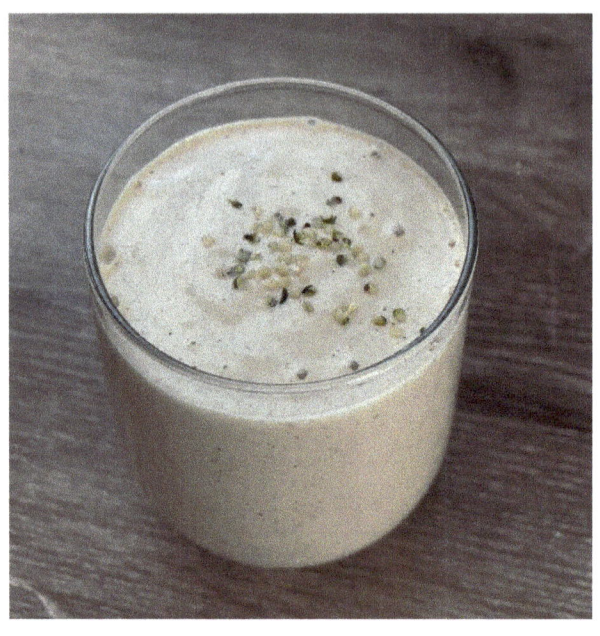

Prep. Time:	Cook Time:	Serves:
5 min	N/A	2

DIRECTIONS

1. Place the cashews in a heat proof dish and cover them in boiling water. Allow this to sit for 10-15 MIN. Drain off the excess liquid and proceed with the recipe.

Traditional ~ Add all the ingredients into a blender and blend for 1 MIN or until you have a smooth mixture.

Thermomix ~ Combine all ingredients into the TM bowl and blitz for 30 SEC / SP 10.

NOTES

If you like a thinner consistency, just add another ¼ cup of coconut water and blend.

INGREDIENTS

- 70g (½ cup) Unsalted Cashews
- 40g (½ cup) Hemp Seeds
- 310g (1 ¼ cups) Organic Coconut Water
- 1 medium Banana
- 5g (1 tsp) Organic Vanilla Bean Paste
- 30g (2 pitted) fresh Medjool Dates
- 20g (1 Tbsp) Nut Butter

BREAKFAST

GREEN GOODNESS SMOOTHIE

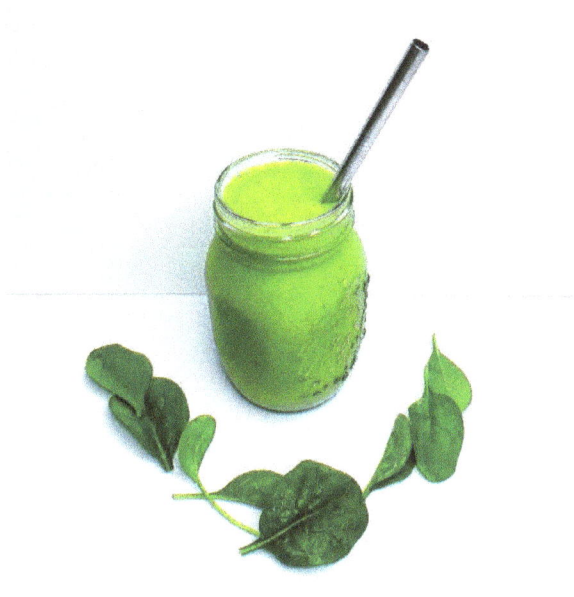

Prep. Time:	Cook Time:	Serves:
5 min	N/A	2

DIRECTIONS

Traditional ~ Add the spinach leaves and liquid into a blender and blend together until there are no large spinach pieces. Add the remaining ingredients and blend until you have a smooth mixture.

Thermomix ~ Add the spinach leaves and liquid into the TM bowl and blitz for 10 SEC / SP 10. Add the remaining ingredients and blitz for 30 SEC / SP 10.

NOTES

You can substitute the banana for ½ a small avocado or leave it out completely.

INGREDIENTS

- 30g (1 cup) Spinach Leaves - tightly packed
- 250g (1 cup) Almond Milk or Coconut Water
- 130g (1 cup) frozen Mango pieces
- 130g (1 cup) frozen Pineapple pieces
- 30g (½) medium Banana
- 10g (1 Tbsp) Hemp Seeds

BREAKFAST

BERRY BLISS SMOOTHIE

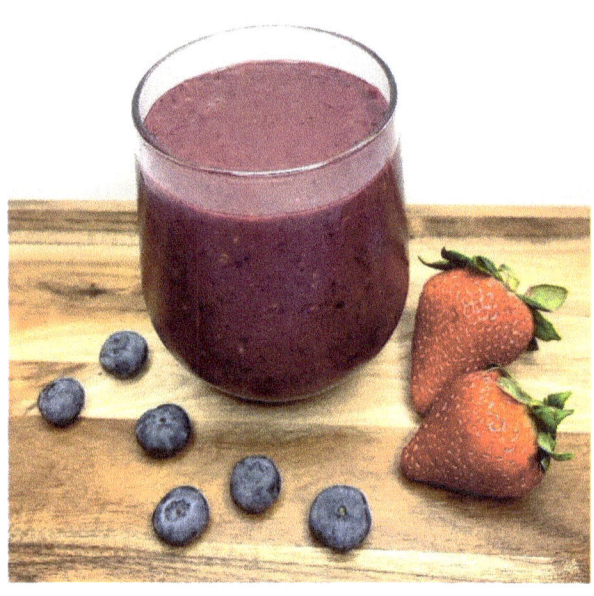

Prep. Time:	Cook Time:	Serves:
5 min	N/A	2

DIRECTIONS

Traditional ~ Add all the ingredients into a blender and blend for 1 MIN or until you have a smooth mixture.

Thermomix ~ Add all the ingredients into the TM bowl and blitz for 30 SEC / SP 10.

NOTES

You can substitute the banana for ½ a medium avocado.

INGREDIENTS

- 250g (1 cup) Almond Milk or Coconut Water
- 130g (1 cup) fresh Organic Strawberry pieces
- 135g (1 cup) frozen Organic Blueberries
- 140g (1 cup) frozen Organic Raspberries
- 150g (1 large) Banana
- 1 scoop Plant-based Berry Protein Powder

DRINKS

CASHEW NUT MILK

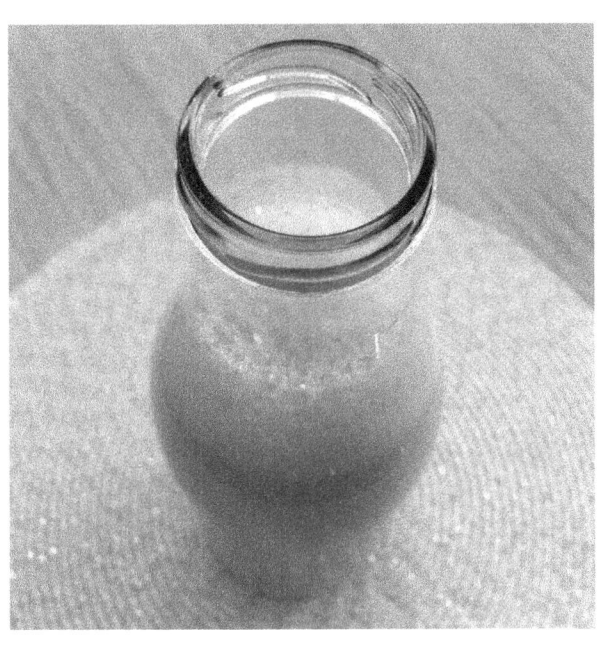

Prep. Time:	Make Time:	Makes:
10 min	5 min	700 ml

DIRECTIONS

1. If time allows, cover and soak your nuts in a bowl of filtered water overnight. Otherwise, tip the cashews and macadamias into a heat proof dish and cover the nuts with boiling water. Allow this to sit for 10-15 MIN.
2. Drain off the excess liquid and proceed with the recipe.

Traditional ~ Using a blender, add the vanilla bean paste and 1 cup of water. Blend together.

Add the drained nuts, plus the remaining 2 cups of water and lecithin granules (if using) and blend for 1 MIN.

Thermomix ~ Add the vanilla bean paste and 1 cup of water into the TM bowl and mix for 10 SEC / SP 4.

Add the drained nuts, plus the remaining 2 cups of water and lecithin granules (if using) to the TM bowl. Blitz for 20 SEC / SP 7.

~~~~~~~~~~~~~~~

Strain the liquid through a nut milk bag into a separate large jug. This helps to separate the milk from the fine nuts. Pour the strained nut milk into a large sealable glass milk bottle and refrigerate.

NOTES

Store in the fridge in an airtight bottle for up to 4 days.

INGREDIENTS

- 150g (1 ¼ cups) Unsalted Cashews
- 50g (⅓ cup) Macadamia Nuts
- 10g (2 tsp) Organic Vanilla Bean Paste
- 740g (3 cups) Filtered Water
- 20g (2 Tbsp) Lecithin Granules (optional – it helps to emulsify)

DRINKS

ALMOND MILK

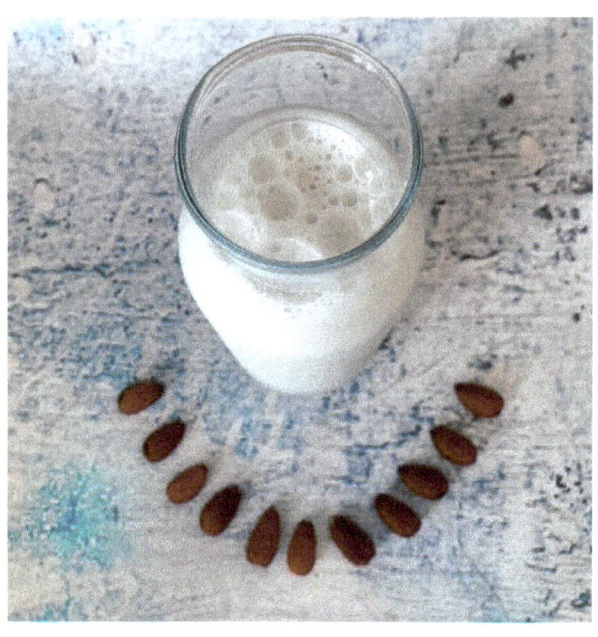

Prep. Time:	Make Time:	Makes:
1 min	5 min	750 ml

DIRECTIONS

1. Place the almonds into a bowl and cover with water. Allow this to sit overnight.
2. Drain off the excess liquid.

Traditional ~ Using a blender, add the drained nuts, water, vanilla bean paste, date and salt. Blend together for 1 MIN.

Thermomix ~ Add the drained nuts, water, vanilla bean paste, date and salt into the TM bowl. Blitz for 1 MIN / SP 10.

~ ~ ~ ~ ~ ~ ~ ~ ~ ~ ~ ~ ~ ~ ~

Strain the liquid through a nut milk bag into a large jug. This helps to separate the milk from the fine nuts. Pour the strained nut milk into a large sealable glass milk bottle and refrigerate.

NOTES

Store in the fridge in an airtight bottle for up to 4 days.

INGREDIENTS

- 150g (1 cup) Natural Almonds
- 740g (3 cups) Filtered Water
- ½ tsp Organic Vanilla Bean Paste
- 18g (1 pitted) fresh Medjool Date
- Pinch of fine Sea Salt

DRINKS

MULLED APPLE JUICE

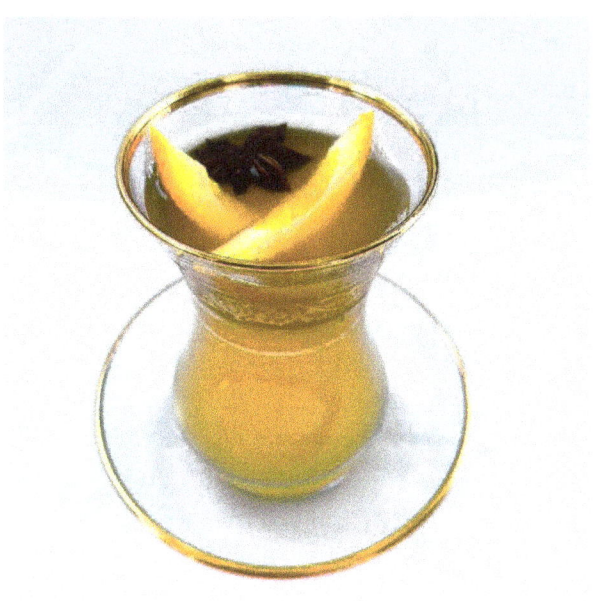

INGREDIENTS

- 1 litre Apple Juice (good quality)
- Thin Strips of Rind from 1 large Orange (keep a few strips aside for serving)
- 1 Cinnamon Quill
- 1-2 Cloves
- 3 Cardamom Pods
- 2 Star Anise + extra for serving
- ¼ tsp ground Nutmeg

Prep. Time: 10 min **Cook Time:** 20 min **Serves:** 4

DIRECTIONS

Traditional ~ Add all the ingredients into a saucepan, cover and bring to the boil. Then simmer for 20 MIN.

Thermomix ~ Add all the ingredients into the TM bowl and cook for 16 MIN / 80°C / SP 1.

~ ~ ~ ~ ~ ~ ~ ~ ~ ~ ~ ~ ~ ~ ~

Strain the liquid through a sieve (or use the TM simmering basket) into a large jug. Pour into glasses and serve immediately.

Garnish each glass with a few strips of orange peel and extra star anise.

NOTES

This is a wonderful drink to serve at Christmas, or in those cooler months to warm you up. It is full of cleansing and anti-inflammatory properties too.

This version is non-alcoholic.

DRINKS

SPICED HOT CHOCOLATE

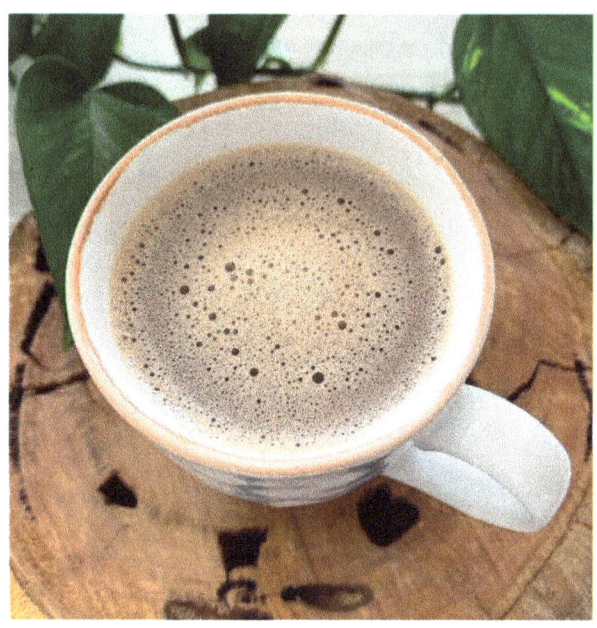

Prep. Time:	Make Time:	Serves:
5 min	5 min	2

DIRECTIONS

Traditional ~ Add all the ingredients (except the essential oil) to a saucepan and heat over a medium–low heat for 5 MIN, using a whisk to stir regularly.

Add the food grade essential oil and whisk until smooth and frothy.

Thermomix ~ Add all the ingredients (except the essential oil) into the TM bowl and heat for 5 MIN / 80°C / SP 1. Add the food grade essential oil and mix for 6 SEC / SP 4.

~ ~ ~ ~ ~ ~ ~ ~ ~ ~ ~ ~ ~ ~ ~

Pour into your favourite cup or mug. Relax, enjoy and take this moment for yourself.

NOTES

Serve immediately.

INGREDIENTS

- 385g (1 ½ cups) Plant-based Milk
- 120g (½ cup) Filtered Water
- 10g (2 Tbsp) Organic Cacao Powder
- 10g (2 tsp) Pure Maple Syrup
- ½ tsp Cinnamon Powder
- ¼ tsp Ginger Powder
- Pinch of Nutmeg
- Pinch of Cayenne Pepper (optional)
- 2 drops Orange Essential Oil (food grade)

DRINKS

TURMERIC TEA

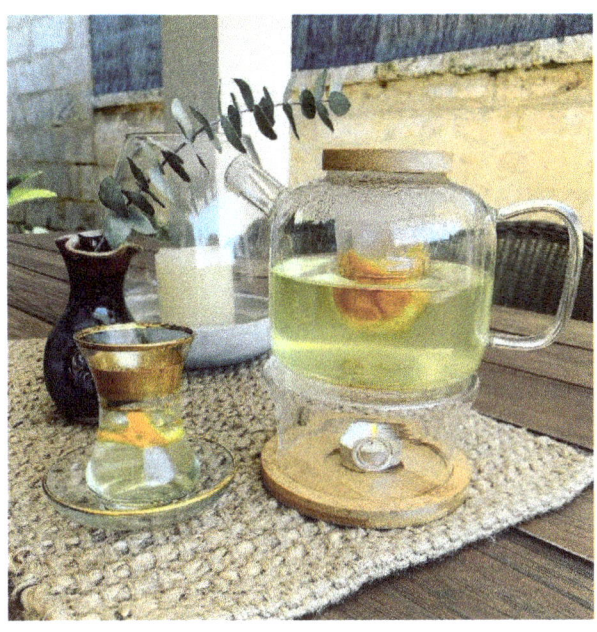

Prep. Time:	Make Time:	Serves:
5 min	5 min	4

DIRECTIONS

Traditional ~ Peel the fresh turmeric and ginger. Add these, plus all remaining ingredients into the strainer of the tea pot as pictured. Allow to brew for 5–10 MIN.

Thermomix ~ Peel the fresh turmeric and ginger. Add these, plus all remaining ingredients into the TM bowl and cook for 5 MIN / 80°C / SP 1.

Use a sieve (or the TM simmering basket) to strain the liquid into a jug. Discard the turmeric, ginger and orange peel.

~ ~ ~ ~ ~ ~ ~ ~ ~ ~ ~ ~ ~ ~

Pour into glasses and serve immediately.

INGREDIENTS

- 730g (3 cups) Boiled Filtered Water
- 2cm piece fresh Turmeric
- 2cm piece fresh Ginger
- 2 pieces of Orange Peel
- 3 tsp Organic Apple Cider Vinegar (with honey if you prefer)

NOTES

This tea is full of immune boosting and anti-inflammatory properties and is also wonderful for gut health.

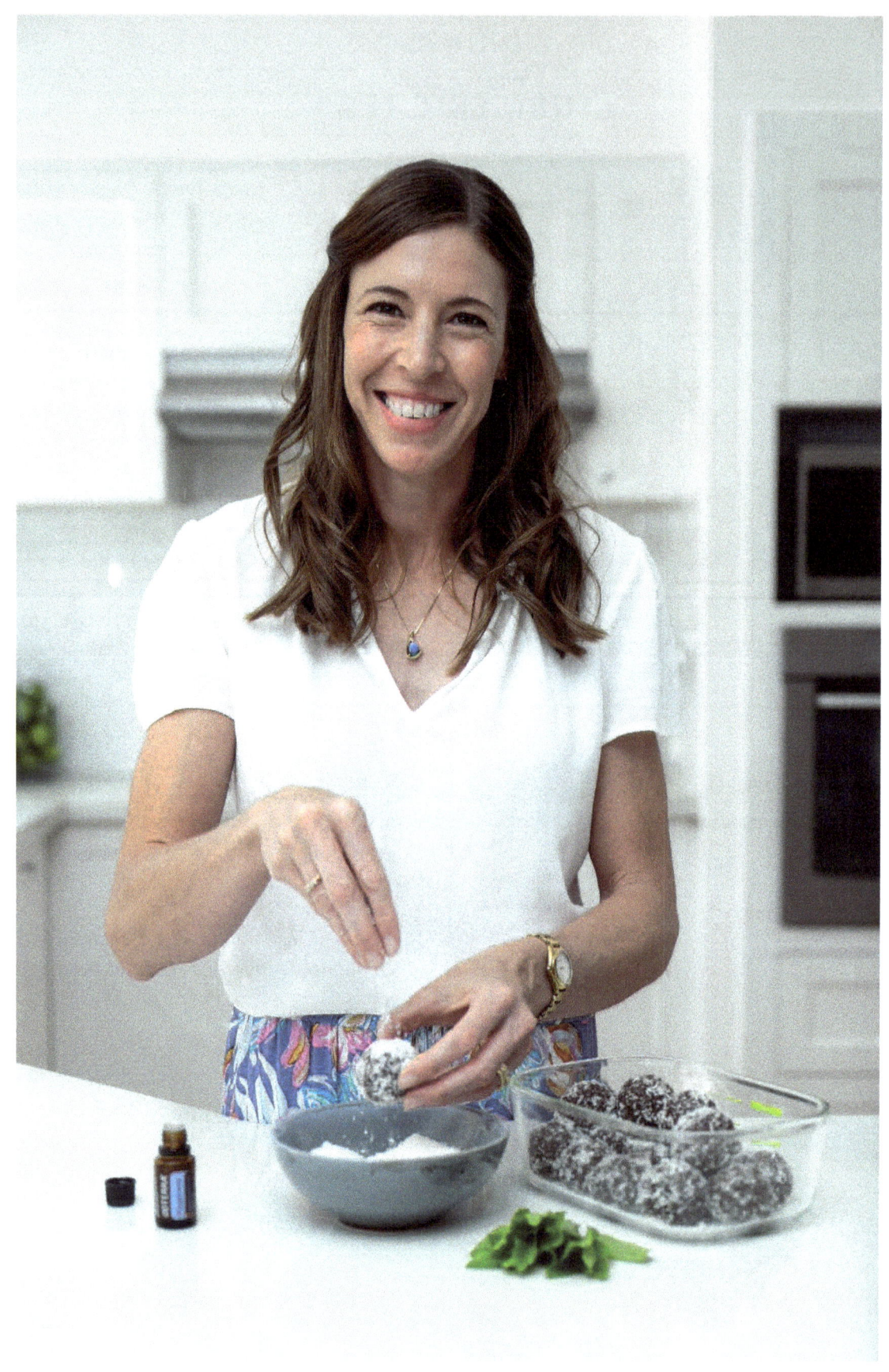

SNACKS

SNACKS

RAW PEANUT BUTTER COOKIES

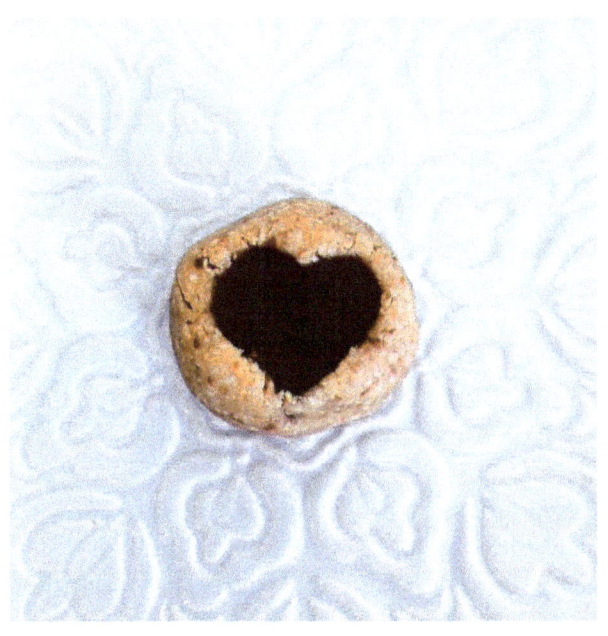

INGREDIENTS

- 80g (1 cup) Organic Rolled Oats
- Pinch of fine Sea Salt
- 125g (7) fresh Pitted Medjool Dates
- 140g (½ cup) Natural Peanut Butter

CHOCOLATE TOPPING

- 15g (1 Tbsp) Organic Coconut Oil
- 5g (1 tsp) Pure Maple Syrup
- 5g (1 Tbsp) Organic Cacao Powder
- Pinch of fine Sea Salt

Prep. Time:	Cook Time:	Makes:
10 min	N/A	10

DIRECTIONS

Traditional ~ Add the oats, salt, dates and peanut butter into a food processor and blitz together until you have a smooth mixture.

Thermomix ~ Add the oats, salt, dates and peanut butter into the TM bowl and blitz together for 10 SEC / SP 9.

~ ~ ~ ~ ~ ~ ~ ~ ~ ~ ~ ~ ~ ~ ~

Line a baking tray with baking paper. Scoop the dough with a spoon and roll into 10 cookie balls. Make an indent / well in the centre of the cookie ball, then place onto the tray and set aside.

CHOCOLATE TOPPING
In a small heat proof bowl, melt the coconut oil in the microwave for 30 SEC. Add the remaining topping ingredients to the melted oil and stir together.

Pour the chocolate topping into the well of each cookie.

Place the tray into the freezer for 10 MIN so the chocolate can set. Once set, remove the tray from the freezer.

NOTES

Store in an airtight container in the fridge for up to 1 week.

SNACKS

MACADAMIA CHOC COOKIES

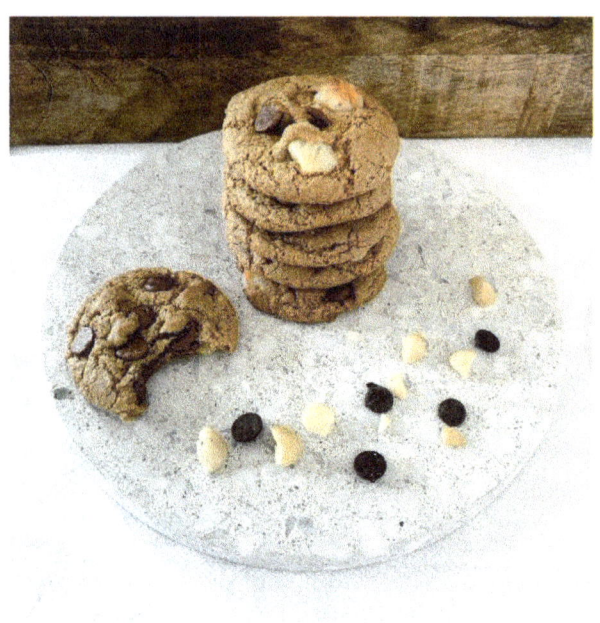

Prep. Time: 5 min
Cook Time: 12 min
Makes: 12

INGREDIENTS

- 60g (¼ cup) Organic Coconut Oil
- 160g (1 cup) Brown Sugar
- 10g (2 tsp) Organic Vanilla Bean Paste
- 65g (¼ cup) Plant-based Milk
- 240g (1 ½ cup) Wholemeal Plain Flour
- ½ tsp Bi-Carb Soda
- 1 tsp Baking Powder
- ¼ tsp fine Sea Salt
- 40g (¼ cup) Macadamia Nuts - roughly chopped
- 40g (¼ cup) Chocolate Chips (dairy free)

DIRECTIONS

Traditional ~ Using a large bowl, mix the coconut oil and brown sugar together. Add the vanilla bean paste, plant-based milk and mix again. Add the flour, bi-carb soda, baking powder and salt. Stir until a cookie batter forms. Gently mix in the macadamia nuts and chocolate chips.

Thermomix ~ Add the coconut oil and brown sugar into the TM bowl. Mix for 10 SEC / SP 4. Scrape down the sides of the bowl and mix again for 10 SEC / SP 4. Add the remaining ingredients except for the nuts and choc chips. Mix for 40 SEC / SP 4. Add the nuts and choc chips and stir for 20 SEC / REVERSE / SP 2.

~ ~ ~ ~ ~ ~ ~ ~ ~ ~ ~ ~ ~ ~ ~

Line 2 baking trays with baking paper. Using a spoon, scoop the mixture and roll into 12 balls. Place each ball onto the tray and slightly flatten each one.

Bake in the oven at 180°C for 12 MIN.

NOTES

Allow to cool completely. Store in an airtight container in the pantry for up to 1 week.

You can leave out the nuts and increase the chocolate chips for a nut free version.

SNACKS

CASHEW SESAME SLICE

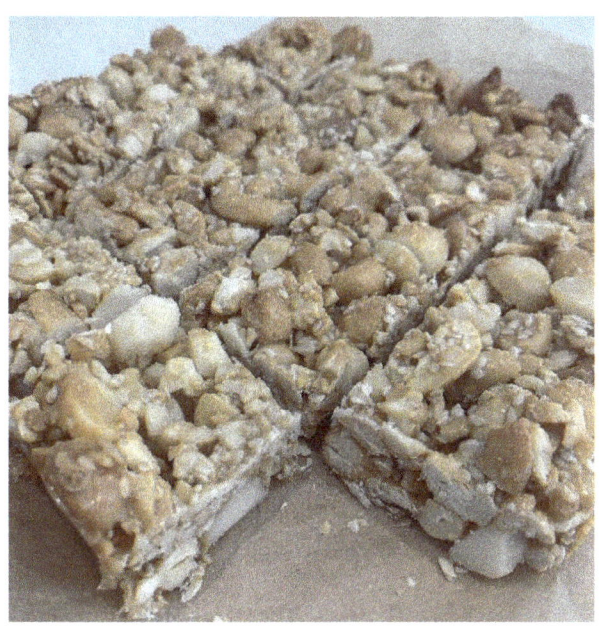

Prep. Time:	Cook Time:	Makes:
5 min	20 min	16

DIRECTIONS

Traditional ~ Add all the ingredients into a large bowl and stir until combined and evenly coated.

Thermomix ~ Add all the ingredients into the TM bowl and mix for 8 SEC / SP 3.

~~~~~~~~~~~~~~~

Line a square slice tray with baking paper and empty the mixture into it. Press the entire slice down firmly with a spatula.

Bake in the oven at 160°C for 20 MIN.

NOTES

Allow to cool completely, then slice into 16 pieces and store in an airtight container in the pantry for up to 1 week.

INGREDIENTS

- 270g (2 cups) Unsalted Cashews
- 100g (¾ cup) Unsalted Macadamia Nuts
- 20g (2 Tbsp) Sesame Seeds
- 80g (¼ cup) Organic Rice Malt Syrup
- 10g (2 tsp) Organic Raw Sugar
- ¼ tsp fine Sea Salt

SNACKS

FRUIT NUT SLICE

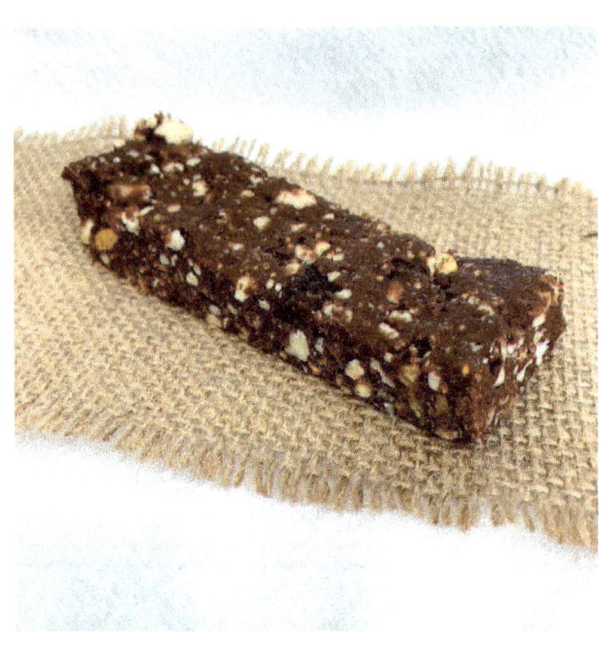

Prep. Time: 10 min
Freeze Time: 1 hr
Makes: 18

DIRECTIONS

Traditional ~ In a food processor, blitz the nuts into little pieces, then add the dried fruit and blitz again. Place all the remaining ingredients into the food processor and blitz until the mixture is combined.

Thermomix ~ Place all the ingredients into the TM bowl and blitz together for 30 SEC / SP 10.

~~~~~~~~~~~~~~~

Line a slice tray with baking paper. Press the mixture into the tray and freeze for 1 HOUR.

Remove from the freezer and slice into bars.

NOTES

Store in an airtight container in the fridge for up to 2 weeks.

INGREDIENTS

- 75g (½ cup) Natural Almonds
- 75g (½ cup) Unsalted Cashews
- 180g (10 pitted) fresh Medjool Dates
- 120g (8) dried Figs
- 35g (¼ cup) Raisins
- 25g (¼ cup) Organic Cacao Powder
- 60g (¼ cup) Organic Coconut Oil

SNACKS

HAZELNUT PROTEIN BALLS

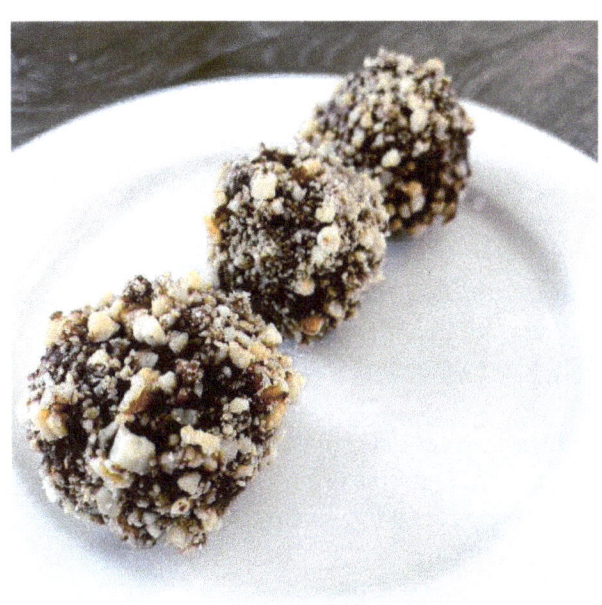

Prep. Time: 15 min **Freeze Time:** 1 hr **Makes:** 18

DIRECTIONS

Traditional ~ Place the nuts into a food processor and blitz together until fine. Add the remaining ingredients for the protein balls and blitz again until the mixture is well combined.

Thermomix ~ Place the nuts into the TM bowl and blitz for 5 SEC / SP 9. Add the remaining ingredients for the protein balls and blitz again for 30 SEC / SP 9.

~ ~ ~ ~ ~ ~ ~ ~ ~ ~ ~ ~ ~ ~ ~

Scoop and roll a small amount of the mixture into balls. Place the balls onto a lined tray. Place the tray into the freezer for up to 1 HOUR to firm up.

DIPPING SAUCE
Traditional ~ Melt the coconut oil in a heat proof bowl in the microwave for 30 SEC. Add in the cacao powder and maple syrup. Stir until combined and set aside.

Thermomix ~ Place the coconut oil, cacao powder and maple syrup into the TM bowl. Melt for 2 MIN / 70°C / SP STIR. Then mix for 5 SEC / SP 5. Pour into a small bowl and set aside.

TO ASSEMBLE
Make the nut crumble by finely chopping the cup of mixed nuts. Place into a bowl and set aside. Remove the protein balls from the freezer. Use a bamboo skewer to hold each ball. Carefully dip each ball into the dipping sauce, followed by a coating of the chopped nuts. Place onto the tray Repeat for each one. Place into the fridge to set.

INGREDIENTS

PROTEIN BALLS

- 130g (1 ¼ cup) Hazelnuts
- 130g (1 cup) Unsalted Cashews
- 160g (9 pitted) fresh Medjool Dates
- 40g (½ cup) Organic Desiccated Coconut
- 55g (½ cup) Organic Cacao Powder
- 40g (2 Tbsp) Pure Maple Syrup
- 15g (1 Tbsp) Organic Coconut Oil

DIPPING SAUCE

- 45g (3 Tbsp) Organic Coconut Oil
- 40g (⅓ cup) Organic Cacao Powder
- 20g (1 Tbsp) Pure Maple Syrup

NUT CRUMBLE TOPPING

- 250g (1 cup) Mixed nuts – I used finely chopped unsalted Cashews and Hazelnuts

NOTES

Store in an airtight container in the fridge for up to 1 week.

SNACKS

BANANA CINNAMON BREAD

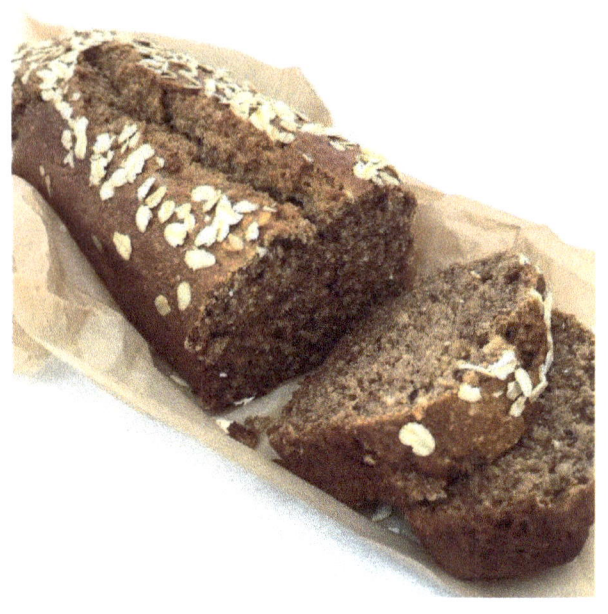

INGREDIENTS

- 350g (3 large) Bananas
- 110g (½ cup) Organic Coconut Oil
- 80g (¼ cup) Pure Maple Syrup
- 5g (1 tsp) Organic Vanilla Bean Paste
- 320g (2 cups) Wholemeal Plain Flour
- 160g (1 cup) Brown Sugar / Coconut Sugar
- 1 tsp ground Cinnamon
- ¼ tsp Ginger Powder
- ½ tsp Baking Soda
- 5g (1 tsp) Baking Powder
- 50g (½ cup) Walnuts (optional)

Prep. Time:	Cook Time:	Makes:
5 min	60 min	12 slices

DIRECTIONS

Traditional ~ In a large bowl, mash the bananas with a fork. Add the remaining wet ingredients and mix until combined, either by hand or with beaters on a medium–low speed.

Scrape down the sides of the bowl. Add in the dry ingredients and stir until combined using the same speed. If adding walnuts, gently stir them through with a spoon.

Thermomix ~ Add the bananas into the TM bowl and mash for 4 SEC / SP 4. Add the remaining wet ingredients and mix for 10 SEC / SP 4. Scrape down the sides of the bowl.

Add the dry ingredients and mix for 40 SEC / SP 4. Add the walnuts (optional) and mix for 8 SEC / REVERSE / SP 4.

~ ~ ~ ~ ~ ~ ~ ~ ~ ~ ~ ~ ~ ~ ~

Line a bread tin with baking paper. Pour the mixture in.

You can either sprinkle the top with some organic rolled oats or slice a banana in half lengthways and lay it on top, for a fancy look.

Bake in the oven at 160°C for 60 MIN.

NOTES

Allow to cool in the tin, before removing. Store in an airtight container in the pantry.

This freezes beautifully, so slice it up once cooled and freeze pieces in an airtight container ready for lunchboxes. It can be stored in the freezer for up to 4 weeks.

SNACKS

ANZAC SLICE

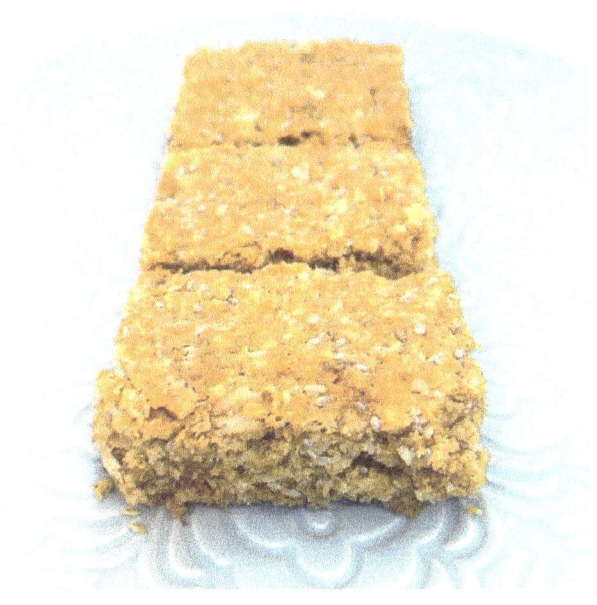

Prep. Time:	Cooking Time:	Makes:
10 min	25 min	24

DIRECTIONS

Traditional ~ Place the coconut oil and golden syrup into a saucepan and melt together over a low heat. Once melted, pour the mixture into a large heat proof mixing bowl. Add the remaining ingredients and stir until combined.

Thermomix ~ Place the coconut oil and golden syrup into the TM bowl and heat for 2 MIN / 90°C / SP 2. Add the remaining ingredients. Mix for 30 SEC / REVERSE / SP 3.

~ ~ ~ ~ ~ ~ ~ ~ ~ ~ ~ ~ ~ ~ ~

Line a baking tin with baking paper and press the mixture firmly into it.

Bake in the oven at 160°C for 25 MIN.

NOTES

Allow to cool completely before slicing.

Slice into bars and store in an airtight container in the pantry for up to 2 weeks.

INGREDIENTS

- 170g (¾ cup) Organic Coconut Oil
- 85g (¼ cup) Golden Syrup
- 15g (1 Tbsp) Boiling Filtered Water
- ½ tsp Bi-Carb Soda
- 75g (⅓ cup) Organic Raw Sugar
- 110g (1 cup) Organic Rolled Oats
- 100g (1 cup) Organic Desiccated Coconut
- 5g (1 tsp) Chia Seeds
- 200g (1 ¼ cups) Wholemeal Plain Flour

SNACKS

CRISPY PEANUT BUTTER BARS

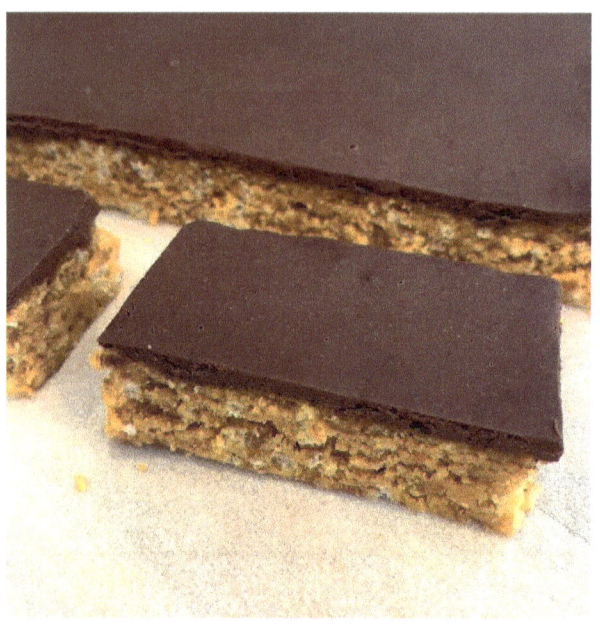

Prep. Time:	Fridge Time:	Makes:
10 min	1 ½ hrs	12

DIRECTIONS

Traditional ~ Blitz the dates in food processor. Tip the date mixture into a large bowl. Add the peanut butter, coconut oil, vanilla bean paste, maple syrup and salt. Mix together. Add the rice bubbles and stir until combined.

Thermomix ~ Add the dates into the TM bowl and blitz for 10 SEC / SP 8. Add the peanut butter, coconut oil, vanilla bean paste, maple syrup and salt. Mix for 10 SEC / SP 4. Add the Rice Bubbles and mix for 40 SEC / REVERSE / SP 3.

~ ~ ~ ~ ~ ~ ~ ~ ~ ~ ~ ~ ~ ~ ~

Line a square baking tray with baking paper. Tip the mixture in and press down firmly. Place in the fridge to set for 1 HOUR.

CHOCOLATE GANACHE TOPPING

Traditional ~ Add the coconut oil and coconut cream into a small saucepan and melt together over a low heat. Then add the maple syrup and cacao powder and whisk together to remove any lumps.

Thermomix ~ In a clean TM bowl, add the coconut cream and coconut oil. Melt for 2 MIN / 70°C / SP 2. Add the maple syrup and cacao powder. Mix for 4 SEC / SP4.

~ ~ ~ ~ ~ ~ ~ ~ ~ ~ ~ ~ ~ ~ ~

Pour the chocolate topping over the slice and return to the fridge to set for 30 MIN. When the topping has set, slice it into bars.

INGREDIENTS

- 180g (10 pitted) fresh Medjool Dates
- 260g (1 cup) Smooth Peanut Butter (good quality)
- 30g (2 Tbsp) Organic Coconut Oil
- 10g (2 tsp) Organic Vanilla Bean Paste
- 40g (2 Tbsp) Pure Maple Syrup
- ¼ tsp fine Sea Salt
- 75g (2 ½ cups) Puffed Rice (Rice Bubbles)

CHOCOLATE GANACHE TOPPING

- 30g (2 Tbsp) Organic Coconut Oil
- 60g (¼ cup) Organic Coconut Cream
- 40g (2 Tbsp) Pure Maple Syrup
- 20g (¼ cup) Organic Cacao Powder

NOTES

Store in an airtight container in the fridge for up to 5 days. Remove from the fridge before serving to allow the ganache to soften slightly.

SNACKS

SALTED CARAMEL RAW BALLS

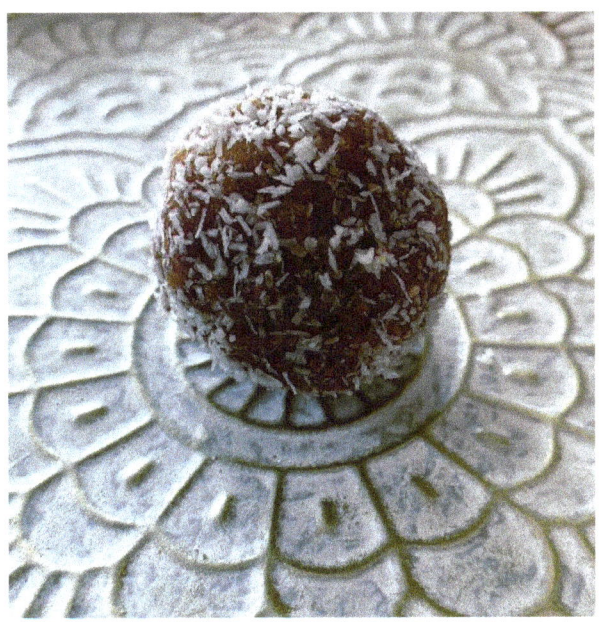

Prep. Time: 5 min
Cook Time: N/A
Makes: 10-14

DIRECTIONS

Traditional ~ Add the flax seeds to a food processor and blitz on high until you have a flour like consistency. Add the remaining ingredients and blitz again until the mixture is well combined.

Thermomix ~ Add the flax seeds into the TM bowl and blitz for 9 SEC / SP 9. Add the remaining ingredients and blitz for 30 SEC / SP 9.

~~~~~~~~~~~~~~~

Scoop out tablespoon size amounts of mixture and roll in the palms of your hands until a ball shape forms. Roll each ball evenly in organic desiccated coconut.

NOTES

When rolling, these can feel a little sticky, but once refrigerated they become the perfect firmness.

Store in an airtight container in the fridge for up to 2 weeks.

INGREDIENTS

- 40g (¼ cup) Flax Seeds
- 160g (9 pitted) fresh Medjool Dates
- 140g (½ cup) Smooth Peanut Butter
- 10g (1 Tbsp) Chia Seeds
- 10g (1 Tbsp) Maca Powder (optional)
- 20g (1 Tbsp) Organic Vanilla Bean Paste
- 20g (1 Tbsp) Pure Maple Syrup
- ½ tsp fine Sea Salt

SERVING

- Organic Desiccated Coconut for rolling the raw balls in

SNACKS

NO BAKE OAT BARS

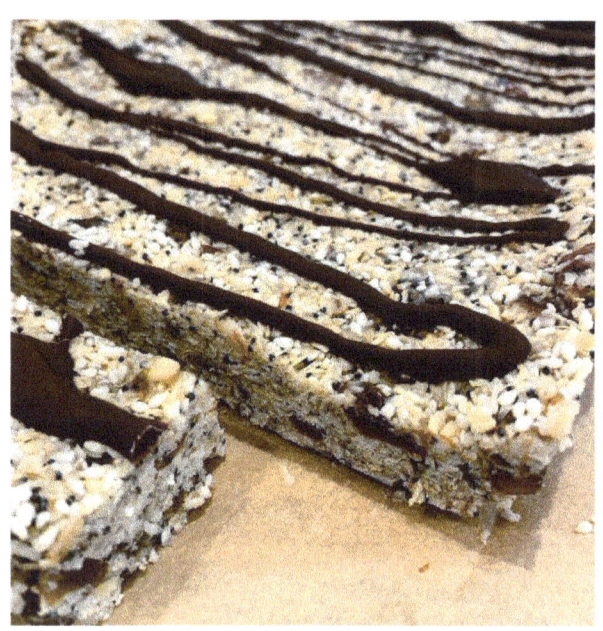

Prep. Time: 10 min
Fridge Time: 2 hrs
Makes: 24

DIRECTIONS

Traditional ~ Add the coconut oil, rice malt syrup and raw sugar to a small saucepan and melt together. Empty this mixture into a large mixing bowl. Add the peanut butter and all the dry ingredients and mix thoroughly until combined.

Thermomix ~ Add the coconut oil, rice malt syrup and raw sugar into the TM bowl for 2 MIN / 70°C / SP 2. Add the peanut butter and dry ingredients and mix for 40 SEC / REVERSE / SP 4.

~ ~ ~ ~ ~ ~ ~ ~ ~ ~ ~ ~ ~ ~ ~

Line a slice tray with baking paper and press the slice into the tin.

CHOCOLATE TOPPING

In a heat proof bowl, add the chocolate chips and coconut oil. Melt together in the microwave for 1 MIN. Drizzle over the top of the slice.

Place the slice into the fridge for 2 HOURS to set.

NOTES

Once set, slice into pieces and store in an airtight container in the fridge for up to 2 weeks.

INGREDIENTS

- 60g (¼ cup) Organic Coconut Oil
- 160g (½ cup) Organic Rice Malt Syrup
- 60g (¼ cup) Organic Raw Sugar
- 75g (¼ cup) Smooth Peanut Butter (good quality)
- 185g (2 cups) Organic Rolled Oats
- 100g (1 ½ cups) Organic Shredded Coconut
- 70g (½ cup) Sesame Seeds
- 20g (2 Tbsp) Poppy Seeds
- 30g (2 Tbsp) Chia Seeds
- 150g (1 cup) Organic Raisins

CHOCOLATE TOPPING

- 50g (¼ cup) dairy free Chocolate Chips
- 1 tsp Organic Coconut Oil

SNACKS

PEPPERMINT PROTEIN BALLS

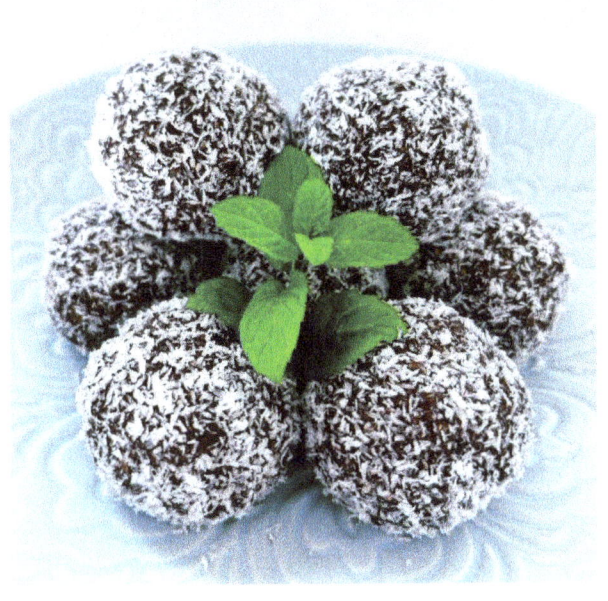

Prep. Time:	Cook Time:	Makes:
5 min	N/A	18

DIRECTIONS

Traditional ~ Add the almonds, sunflower kernels and chia seeds into a food processor and blitz together until you have a fine crumb. Add the remaining ingredients and the food grade essential oil and blitz again for 1 MIN or until combined.

Thermomix ~ Add the almonds, sunflower kernels and chia seeds into the TM bowl and blitz for 10 SEC / SP 10. Add the remaining ingredients and the food grade essential oil and blitz for 30 SEC / SP 9.

~ ~ ~ ~ ~ ~ ~ ~ ~ ~ ~ ~ ~ ~ ~

Scoop out tablespoon size amounts of mixture and roll in the palms of your hands until a ball shape forms. Roll each ball in organic desiccated coconut.

INGREDIENTS

- 225g (1 ½ cups) Natural Almonds
- 45g (⅓ cup) Sunflower Kernels
- 20g (2 Tbsp) Chia Seeds
- 55g (¾ cup) Organic Shredded Coconut
- 75g (¾ cup) Organic Cacao Powder
- 120g (⅓ cup) Organic Rice Malt Syrup
- 145g (8 pitted) fresh Medjool Dates
- 8 drops Peppermint Essential Oil (food grade)

SERVING

- Organic Desiccated Coconut for rolling the raw balls in

NOTES

*If the mixture is a bit dry, add either 1 Tbsp of Rice Malt Syrup or another date (some dates are drier than others and we want those big soft ones), so that the mixture holds together.

You can also replace the Natural Almonds with 2 cups loosely packed Almond Meal.

Store in an airtight container in the pantry for up to 3 weeks.

SNACKS

NUT FREE BLISS BALLS

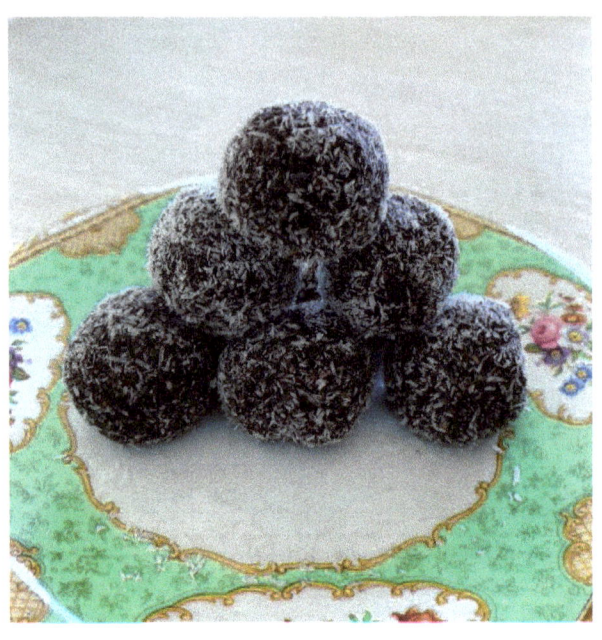

INGREDIENTS

- 50g (⅓ cup) Sunflower Kernels
- 70g (½ cup) Hemp Seeds
- 55g (¾ cup) Organic Shredded Coconut
- 110g (6 pitted) fresh Medjool Dates
- 30g (⅓ cup) Organic Cacao Powder
- 40g (2 Tbsp) Organic Rice Malt Syrup
- 5g (1 tsp) Organic Vanilla Bean Paste
- 6 drops Peppermint Essential Oil (food grade) - optional

SERVING

- Organic Desiccated Coconut for rolling the raw balls in

Prep. Time:	Cook Time:	Makes:
5 min	N/A	10

DIRECTIONS

Traditional ~ Add the sunflower kernels, hemp seeds and shredded coconut into a food processor and blitz together. Add the dates and blitz again. Add the remaining ingredients (including the food grade essential oil) and blitz until well combined.

Thermomix ~ Add the sunflower kernels, hemp seeds and shredded coconut into the TM bowl and blitz for 5 SEC / SP 10. Add the dates and the remaining ingredients (including the food grade essential oil) and blitz for 9 SEC / SP 9.

~ ~ ~ ~ ~ ~ ~ ~ ~ ~ ~ ~ ~ ~ ~

Scoop out tablespoon size amounts of mixture and roll in the palms of your hands until a ball shape forms. Roll each ball in organic desiccated coconut.

NOTES

Store in an airtight container in the fridge for up to 3 weeks.

SNACKS

THE BIG COOKIE

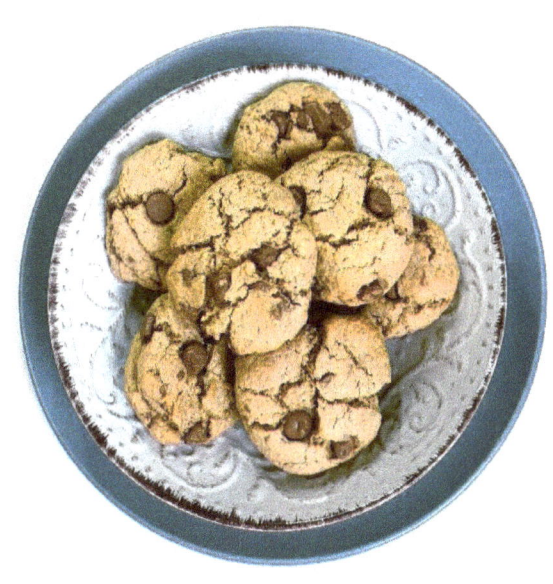

Prep. Time: 10 min   Cook Time: 15 min   Makes: 16

DIRECTIONS

Traditional ~ In a large bowl, beat together the coconut oil, brown sugar and vanilla bean paste. Add the coconut cream and apple sauce. Mix until combined and set aside.

In a separate bowl, add the flour, bi-carb soda, baking powder and salt. Mix then add this mixture into the wet ingredients bowl and beat for 2 MIN. Fold in the chocolate chips.

Thermomix ~ Place the coconut oil, brown sugar and vanilla paste into the TM bowl and mix for 2 MIN / SP 3.

Add the coconut cream, apple sauce, flour, bi-carb soda, baking powder and salt. Mix for 40 SEC / SP 4. Scrape down the sides of the bowl. Mix again for 40 SEC / SP 4.

Add the chocolate chips and stir for 15 SEC / REVERSE / SP 3.

~ ~ ~ ~ ~ ~ ~ ~ ~ ~ ~ ~ ~ ~ ~

Line 2 baking trays with baking paper. Scoop out tablespoons of the cookie mixture and roll into balls, then flatten each one slightly.

Bake in the oven at 180°C for 15 MIN.

INGREDIENTS

- 110g (½ cup) Organic Coconut Oil
- 200g (1 ¼ cup) Brown Sugar
- 10g (2 tsp) Organic Vanilla Bean Paste
- 60g (¼ cup) Organic Coconut Cream
- 60g (¼ cup) Apple Sauce
- 390g (2 ½ cups) Wholemeal Plain Flour
- ½ tsp Bi-Carb Soda
- 5g (1 tsp) Baking Powder
- ½ tsp fine Sea Salt
- 130g (¾ cup) dairy free Chocolate Chips

NOTES

Store in an airtight container in the pantry for up to 2 weeks.

SNACKS

PEANUT BUTTER BLISS BALLS

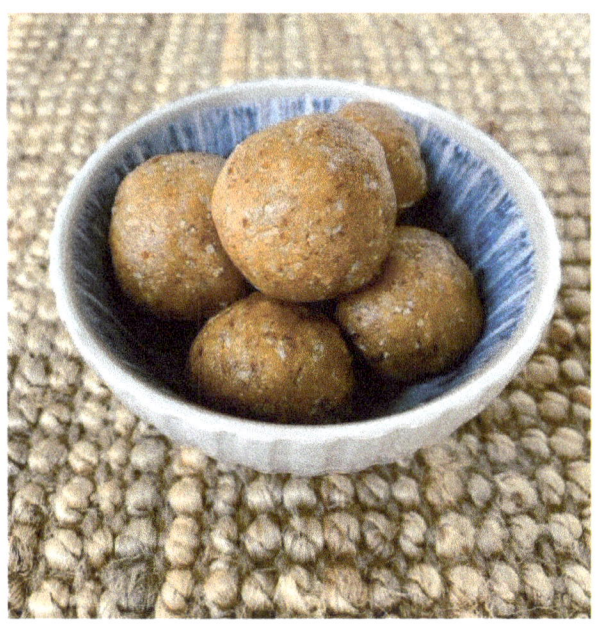

Prep. Time:	Cook Time:	Makes:
5 min	N/A	10

DIRECTIONS

Traditional ~ Add all the ingredients into a food processor and blitz until combined.

Thermomix ~ Add all the ingredients into the TM bowl and blitz for 15 SEC / SP 9.

~~~~~~~~~~~~~~~

Scoop out tablespoon size amounts of mixture and roll in the palms of your hands until a ball shape forms.

INGREDIENTS

- 145g (8 pitted) fresh Medjool Dates
- 100g (1 cup) Almond Meal
- 35g (½ cup) Organic Shredded Coconut
- 45g (3 Tbsp) Smooth Peanut Butter – good quality
- 5g (1 tsp) Organic Vanilla Bean Paste
- ¼ tsp fine Sea Salt

NOTES

Store in an airtight container in the fridge for up to 2 weeks.

SNACKS

LIME BLISS BALLS

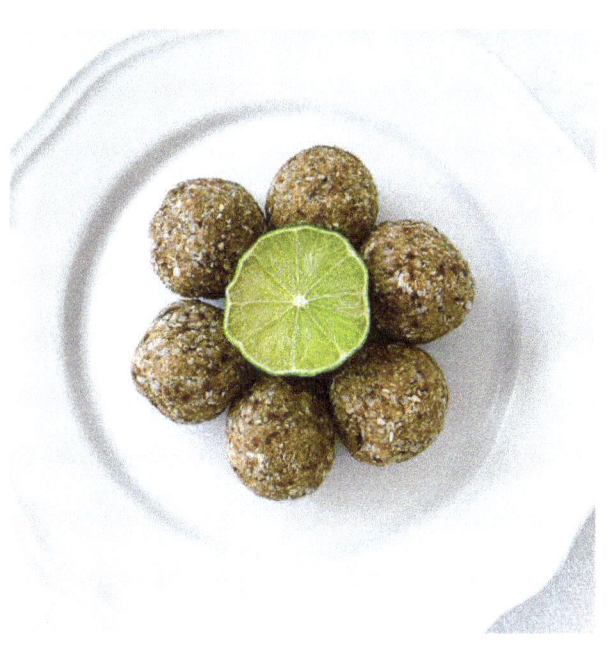

Prep. Time: 5 min
Cook Time: N/A
Makes: 10

DIRECTIONS

Traditional ~ Place all the ingredients into a food processor and blitz together until completely combined.

Thermomix ~ Place all the ingredients into the TM bowl and blitz for 9 SEC / SP 9.

~ ~ ~ ~ ~ ~ ~ ~ ~ ~ ~ ~ ~ ~ ~

Scoop out tablespoon size amounts of mixture and roll in the palms of your hands until a ball shape forms.

NOTES

Store in an airtight container in the fridge for up to 2 weeks.

INGREDIENTS

- 145g (8 pitted) fresh Medjool Dates
- 50g (⅓ cup) Natural Almonds
- 90g (1 cup) Organic Rolled Oats
- Juice of 1 fresh Lime
- 5 drops Lime Essential Oil (food grade) or 1 tsp Lime Zest
- 15g (3 Tbsp) Organic Shredded Coconut

SNACKS

RAW FUDGY BROWNIE

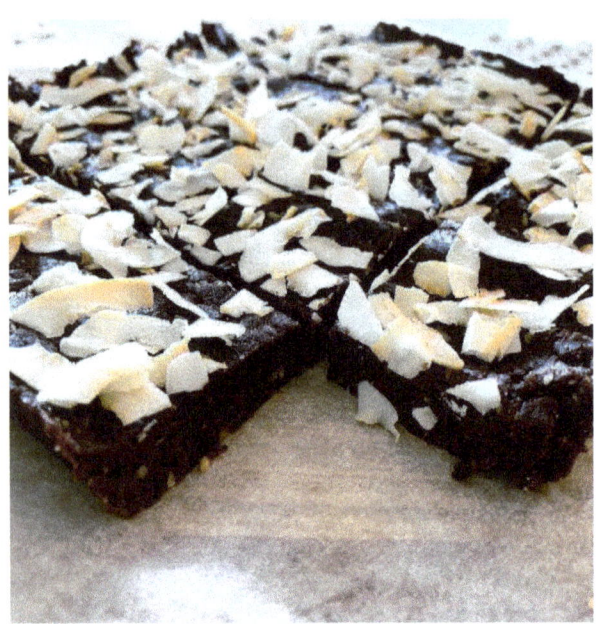

Prep. Time:	Fridge Time:	Makes:
5 min	2 hrs	16

DIRECTIONS

Traditional ~ Blitz the almonds on a high speed in a food processor. Add all the remaining ingredients (except the coconut flakes) and blitz again until well combined.

Thermomix ~ Place the almonds into the TM bowl and blitz for 10 SEC / SP 9. Add all the remaining ingredients (except the coconut flakes) and blitz for 20 SEC / SP 8.

~ ~ ~ ~ ~ ~ ~ ~ ~ ~ ~ ~ ~ ~ ~

Line a baking tray with baking paper and press the brownie mix firmly into the lined tray.

Lightly toast the coconut flakes in a dry frypan for 2 MIN, stirring regularly. Sprinkle the toasted coconut flakes on top of the brownie, gently pressing them in. Place the brownie tray in the fridge for 2 HOURS to set.

NOTES

Once set, remove from the lined tray and slice into pieces.

Store in an airtight container in the pantry for up to 1 week.

INGREDIENTS

- 170g (1 cup) Natural Almonds
- 60g (½ cup) Organic Cacao Powder
- 270g (15 pitted) fresh Medjool Dates
- 15g (1 Tbsp) Brown Sugar
- 20g (1 Tbsp) Pure Maple Syrup
- 40g (2 ½ Tbsp) Organic Coconut Oil
- 40g (⅓ cup) Walnuts

TOPPING

- 15g (⅓ cup) Coconut Flakes (for sprinkling over the brownie)

SNACKS

MUESLI BARS

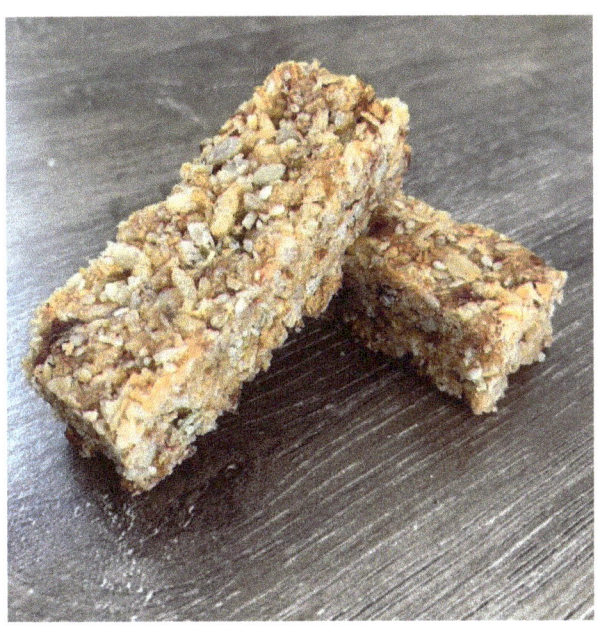

INGREDIENTS

- 35g (¼ cup) Pepitas
- 35g (¼ cup) Sunflower Kernels
- 145g (8 pitted) fresh Medjool Dates
- 100g (½ cup) Organic Raw Sugar
- 90g (¼ cup) Organic Rice Malt Syrup
- 110g (½ cup) Organic Coconut Oil
- 20g (1 Tbsp) Pure Maple Syrup
- 90g (1 cup) Organic Rolled Oats
- 85g (2 ½ cups) Puffed Rice (Rice Bubbles)
- 35g (¼ cup) Sesame Seeds
- 40g (½ cup) Organic Shredded Coconut

Prep. Time:	Cooking Time:	Makes:
10 min	15 min	16

DIRECTIONS

Traditional ~ Roughly chop the pepitas, sunflower kernels and dates. Empty the chopped contents into a bowl and set aside.

Add the sugar and rice malt syrup into a small saucepan. Stir frequently over a medium heat until melted. Add the coconut oil and stir until combined. Remove from the heat and pour into a large mixing bowl.

Add all the remaining ingredients into the mixing bowl (including the seed and date mix) and stir together thoroughly.

Thermomix ~ Place the pepitas, sunflower kernels and dates into the TM bowl and chop for 8 SEC / SP 6. Empty into a separate bowl and set aside.

Add the sugar and rice malt syrup to the TM bowl and melt for 3 MIN / 100°C / SP 1. Add the coconut oil and mix for 4 SEC / SP 4.

Add all the remaining ingredients to the TM bowl, plus the seed and date mix. Mix for 40 SEC / REVERSE / SP 3.

~ ~ ~ ~ ~ ~ ~ ~ ~ ~ ~ ~ ~ ~

Line a slice baking tray with baking paper and press the mixture firmly into the tin.

Bake in the oven at 180°C for 15 MIN.

NOTES

Let it cool in the tray completely before slicing it. Store in an airtight container in the pantry for up to 2 weeks.

SNACKS

CHOC CHIP BLISS BALLS (AND COOKIES)

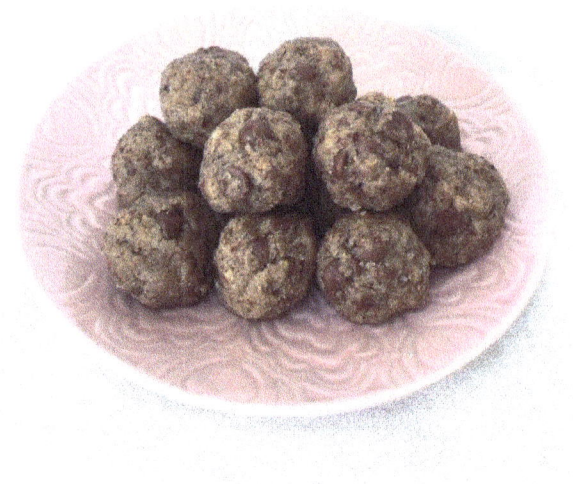

Prep. Time:	Cook Time:	Makes:
5 min	N/A	12

DIRECTIONS

Traditional ~ Using a food processor, add the almonds and blitz until you have a fine crumb consistency. Add the dates, salt, vanilla paste and coconut oil and blitz together until the mixture begins to come together. Empty the mixture into a bowl. Add the chocolate chips and stir through.

Thermomix ~ Add the almonds into the TM bowl and blitz for 6 SEC / SP 9. Add the dates, salt, vanilla paste and coconut oil into the TM bowl. Blitz for 30 SEC / SP 9. Add the chocolate chips and mix for 10 SEC / REVERSE / SP 4.

~ ~ ~ ~ ~ ~ ~ ~ ~ ~ ~ ~ ~ ~ ~

Scoop out tablespoon size amounts of mixture and roll in the palms of your hands until a ball shape forms.

TO MAKE COOKIES
Flatten each bliss ball slightly, then place on a baking tray with baking paper.

Bake in the oven at 180°C for 10 MIN.

NOTES

Store in an airtight container in the fridge (for the bliss balls and in the pantry for the cookies) for up to 2 weeks.

*For a nut free bliss ball lunch box option, substitute the almond meal, for rolled oats (grounded), then add 2 extra dates and triple the vanilla bean paste and coconut oil.

INGREDIENTS

- 225g (1 ½ cups) Natural Almonds OR 2 cups loosely packed Almond Meal
- 125g (7 pitted) fresh Medjool Dates
- ¼ tsp fine Sea Salt
- 5g (1 tsp) Organic Vanilla Bean Paste
- 15g (1 Tbsp) Organic Coconut Oil
- 70g (⅓ cup) Chocolate Chips - dairy free

SNACKS

RAW ORANGE ALMOND SLICE

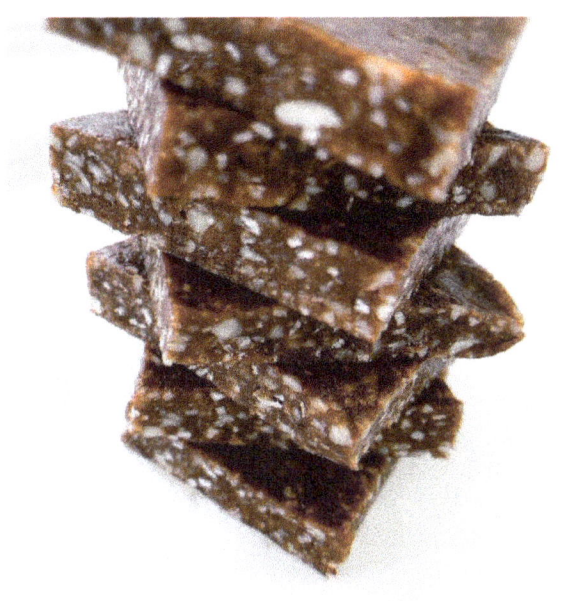

Prep. Time:	Freeze Time:	Makes:
10 min	3 hrs	24

DIRECTIONS

Traditional ~ Add the dates and almonds to a food processor and blitz together.

Empty into a large bowl. Add all the remaining ingredients and mix until combined.

Thermomix ~ Add the dates and almonds into the TM bowl and blitz for 10 SEC / SP 10.

Scrape down the sides of the bowl. Add all the remaining ingredients and mix for 10 SEC / SP 6.

~ ~ ~ ~ ~ ~ ~ ~ ~ ~ ~ ~ ~ ~ ~

Line a square baking tin with baking paper, then press the mixture firmly into the tin. Place into the fridge for 3 HOURS to set, then slice into pieces to serve.

NOTES

Store in an airtight container in the fridge for up to 2 weeks.

INGREDIENTS

- 215g (12 pitted) fresh Medjool Dates
- 150g (1 cup) Natural Almonds
- 15g (3 Tbsp) Organic Cacao Powder
- 10g (2 tsp) Organic Vanilla Bean Paste
- 20g (1 Tbsp) Organic Rice Malt Syrup
- 15g (1 Tbsp) Organic Coconut Oil
- 40g (½ cup) Organic Shredded Coconut
- 10 drops Orange Essential Oil (food grade) or 1 tsp Orange Rind

SNACKS

CARROT WALNUT BREAD

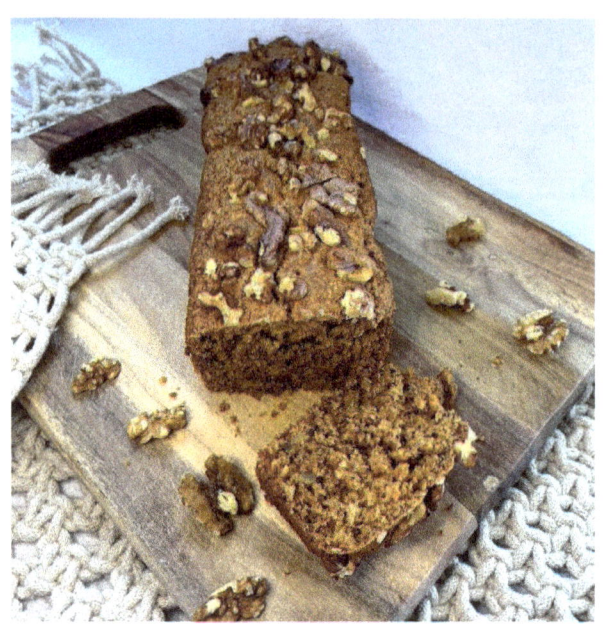

Prep. Time: 15 min
Cook Time: 40 min
Makes: 12

DIRECTIONS

1. Prepare the flax egg by combining 1 Tbsp of flax meal (ground flax seeds) with 2 ½ Tbsp filtered water. Allow this to sit for 5 minutes to thicken.

Traditional ~ Peel and grate the carrot and set aside. Roughly chop the walnuts and set aside. Add all the dry ingredients into a bowl and mix until combined. In a separate bowl add the apple sauce, maple syrup, olive oil, flax egg and grated carrot. Stir to combine. Tip the wet ingredients into the dry ingredients and stir together. Fold through the roughly chopped walnuts.

Thermomix ~ Add the walnuts into the TM bowl. Chop for 4 SEC / SP 4. Empty into a small bowl and set aside. Peel and roughly chop the carrot. Add to the TM bowl and chop for 4 SEC / SP 6. Scrape down the sides of the bowl. Add all the remaining ingredients into the TM bowl, including the flax egg and chopped walnuts. Mix for 40 SEC / REVERSE / SP 4.

~ ~ ~ ~ ~ ~ ~ ~ ~ ~ ~ ~ ~ ~ ~

Line a loaf tin with baking paper. Pour the bread mixture in. Sprinkle the top with the extra chopped walnuts.

Place in the oven and bake at 180°C for 40 MIN.

INGREDIENTS

- 1 Flax Egg
- 160g (1 cup) Wholemeal Plain Flour
- 1 tsp Bi-Carb Soda
- 1 tsp Baking Powder
- ½ tsp fine Sea Salt
- ½ tsp Cinnamon Powder
- 80g (⅔ cup) Organic Rolled Oats
- 80g (⅓ cup) Organic Raw Sugar
- 125g (½ cup) Apple Sauce
- 80g (¼ cup) Pure Maple Syrup
- 55g (¼ cup) Olive Oil
- 50g (½ cup) Walnuts
- 100g (1 medium) Carrot

TOPPING

- 50g (½ cup) Walnuts for the topping – roughly chopped

NOTES

Allow the bread to cool in the tin completely before emptying it onto a cooling rack.

Store in an airtight container in the pantry for up to 1 week.

SNACKS

NOURISH SLICE

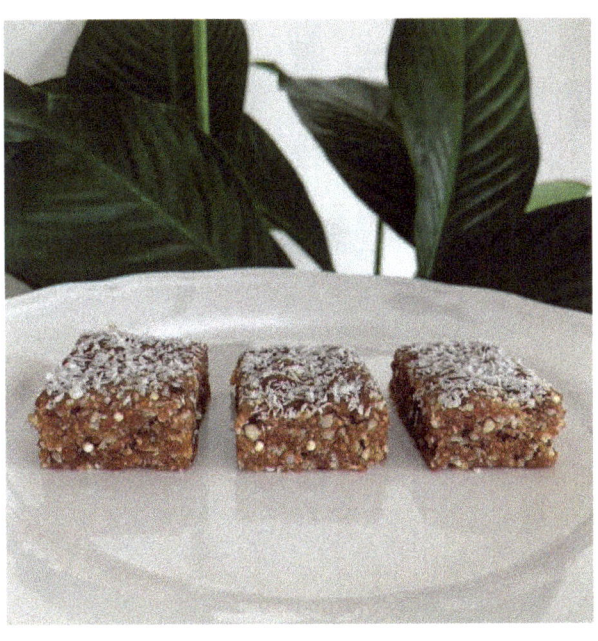

Prep. Time:	Fridge Time:	Makes:
10 min	2 hrs	24

DIRECTIONS

Traditional ~ Place the walnuts, almonds, cashews, brazil nuts, buckwheat, shredded coconut, sunflower kernels, sesame seeds, flax seeds and quinoa into a food processor and blitz together until you have a crumb consistency. Empty this mix into a separate large bowl and set aside.

Blitz together the dates, figs, sultanas and goji berries in the food processor. Then tip the fruit mix into the nut mix. Add the walnut oil, coconut oil, beetroot powder and salt. Stir together until it is combined.

Thermomix ~ Place the walnuts, almonds, cashews, brazil nuts, buckwheat, shredded coconut, sunflower kernels, sesame seeds, flax seeds and quinoa into the TM bowl. Chop for 7 SEC / SP 7. Empty this nut mix into a separate bowl and set aside.

Add the dates, figs, sultanas and goji berries into the TM bowl and blitz for 9 SEC / SP 9. Tip the nut mix into the TM bowl, then add the walnut oil, coconut oil, beetroot powder and salt. Mix for 40 SEC / SP 4.

~ ~ ~ ~ ~ ~ ~ ~ ~ ~ ~ ~ ~ ~ ~

Line a square baking tray with baking paper. Press the mixture firmly into the tray. Sprinkle with organic desiccated coconut (if desired).

Place in the fridge for 2 HOURS. Once firm cut into bite size pieces.

NOTES

Store in an airtight container in the fridge for up to 3 weeks.

INGREDIENTS

- 50g (½ cup) Unsalted Walnuts
- 75g (½ cup) Natural Almonds
- 65g (½ cup) Unsalted Cashews
- 35g (¼ cup) Brazil Nuts
- 50g (¼ cup) Organic Buckwheat
- 20g (¼ cup) Organic Shredded Coconut
- 15g (2 Tbsp) Sunflower Kernels
- 10g (1 Tbsp) Sesame Seeds
- 10g (1 Tbsp) Flax Seeds
- 15g (1 Tbsp) Quinoa
- 180g (10 pitted) fresh Medjool Dates
- 55g (5) Organic Dried Figs
- 80g (½ cup) Organic Sultanas
- 30g (¼ cup) Goji Berries
- 5g (1 tsp) Walnut Oil
- 10g (2 tsp) Beetroot Powder
- ¼ tsp fine Sea Salt

TOPPING

- Organic Desiccated Coconut

SNACKS

MUD MUFFINS

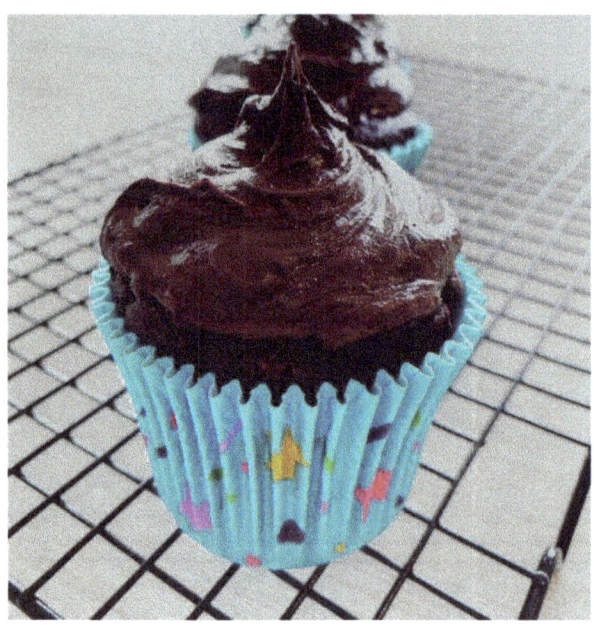

Prep. Time: 10 min
Cook Time: 22 min
Makes: 8

DIRECTIONS

Traditional ~ Add your dry ingredients into a large mixing bowl and stir together. Add the wet ingredients into the bowl and mix until combined.

Thermomix ~ Add all the ingredients into the TM bowl and mix for 1 MIN 30 SEC / SP 7.

~ ~ ~ ~ ~ ~ ~ ~ ~ ~ ~ ~ ~ ~

Scoop the mixture into a lined muffin tray.

Bake in the oven at 180°C for 22 MIN.

Allow the muffins to cool completely before icing.

~ ~ ~ ~ ~ ~ ~ ~ ~ ~ ~ ~ ~ ~

CHOCOLATE ICING

Traditional ~ Combine all the icing ingredients into a bowl and mix with beaters until it is thick and creamy.

Thermomix ~ Add all the icing ingredients into a clean TM bowl and mix for 30 SEC / SP 9.

~ ~ ~ ~ ~ ~ ~ ~ ~ ~ ~ ~ ~ ~

Once the muffins have cooled completely, smooth the icing over the top of each.

NOTES

Store in an airtight container in the fridge for up to 3 days.

INGREDIENTS

- 160g (1 cup) Wholemeal Plain Flour
- 150g (1 ½ cups) Organic Cacao Powder
- 15g (1 Tbsp) Baking Powder
- 80g (½ cup) Brown Sugar
- 150g (½ cup) Pure Maple Syrup
- 330g (1 ⅓ cups) Plant-based Milk
- 10g (2 tsp) Organic Vanilla Bean Paste

CHOCOLATE ICING

- 100g (¾ cup) Icing Sugar
- 70g (¾ cup) Organic Cacao Powder
- 40g (2 Tbsp) Coconut Cream – solid part only
- 45g (3 Tbsp) Plant-based Milk
- ½ tsp Organic Vanilla Bean Paste

SNACKS

SWEET N SALTY NUTS

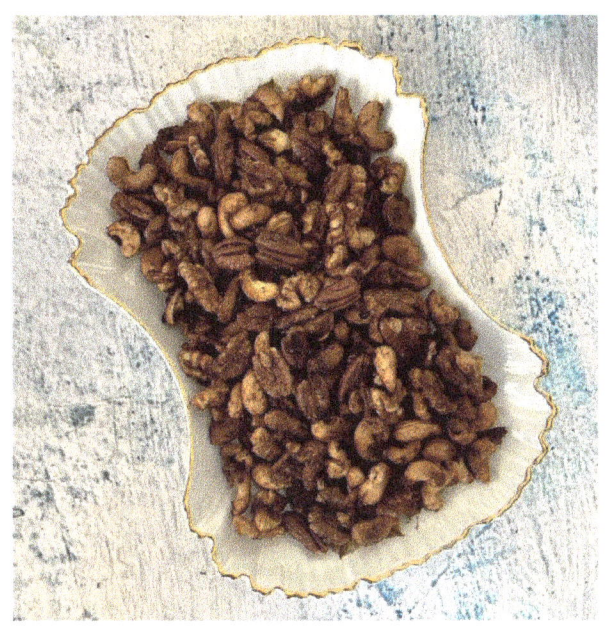

Prep. Time:	Cook Time:	Makes:
2 min	15 min	500g

DIRECTIONS

Traditional ~ Place all the ingredients (except the coconut sugar) into a large mixing bowl and stir to combine.

Thermomix ~ Place all the ingredients (except the coconut sugar) into the TM bowl. Mix for 10 SEC / REVERSE / SP 2.

~ ~ ~ ~ ~ ~ ~ ~ ~ ~ ~ ~ ~ ~ ~

Line a baking tray with baking paper, then empty the nut mixture onto the tray, spreading it out evenly.

Bake in the oven at 180°C for 12-15 MIN, stirring halfway.

Once removed from the oven, sprinkle the coconut sugar over the top.

NOTES

Allow to cool completely then store in an airtight container in the pantry for up to 2 weeks or in the freezer for up to 1 month.

INGREDIENTS

- 150g (1 ⅓ cups) Unsalted Pecans
- 150g (1 ⅓ cup) Unsalted Walnuts
- 190g (1 ⅓ cup) Unsalted Cashews
- 80g (4 Tbsp) Pure Maple Syrup
- 30g (2 Tbsp) Organic Coconut Oil (melted)
- 1 tsp ground Cumin
- 1 tsp fine Sea Salt
- ½ tsp Garlic Powder
- ¼ tsp Onion Powder
- pinch Cayenne Pepper Powder
- 10g (1 Tbsp) Coconut Sugar

SNACKS

KALE CHIPS

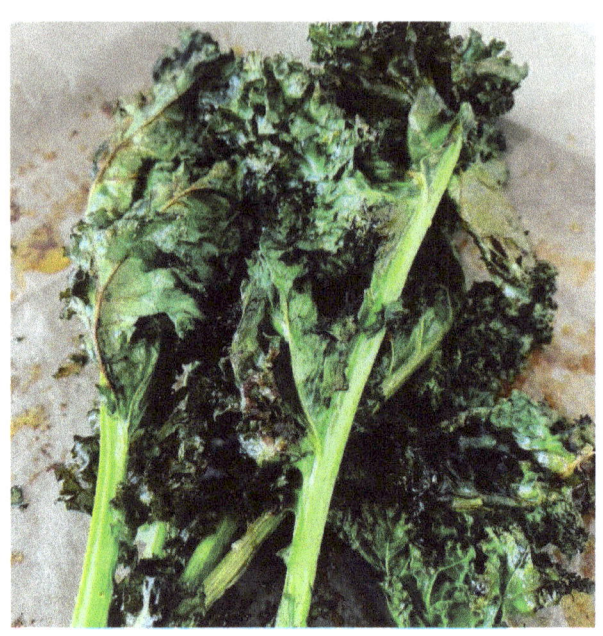

Prep. Time:	Cook Time:	Serves:
10 min	20 min	4

DIRECTIONS – Traditional Only

Traditional ~ Wash and pat dry the kale.

Melt the coconut oil in a small heat proof bowl in the microwave for 30 SEC. Add the spices and salt to the melted oil and stir together.

~ ~ ~ ~ ~ ~ ~ ~ ~ ~ ~ ~ ~ ~ ~

Line a baking tray with baking paper. Place the kale leaves evenly onto the tray and drizzle the spice mix over the top. Gently toss the leaves around, making sure they are evenly coated.

Bake in the oven at 180°C for 20 MIN.

NOTES

Allow to cool slightly before eating.

INGREDIENTS

- 1 Bunch of Fresh Kale
- 30g (2 Tbsp) Organic Coconut Oil - melted
- ¼ tsp Garlic Powder
- ¼ tsp Onion Salt
- ¼ tsp ground Paprika
- ¼ tsp ground Cumin
- ¼ tsp fine Sea Salt

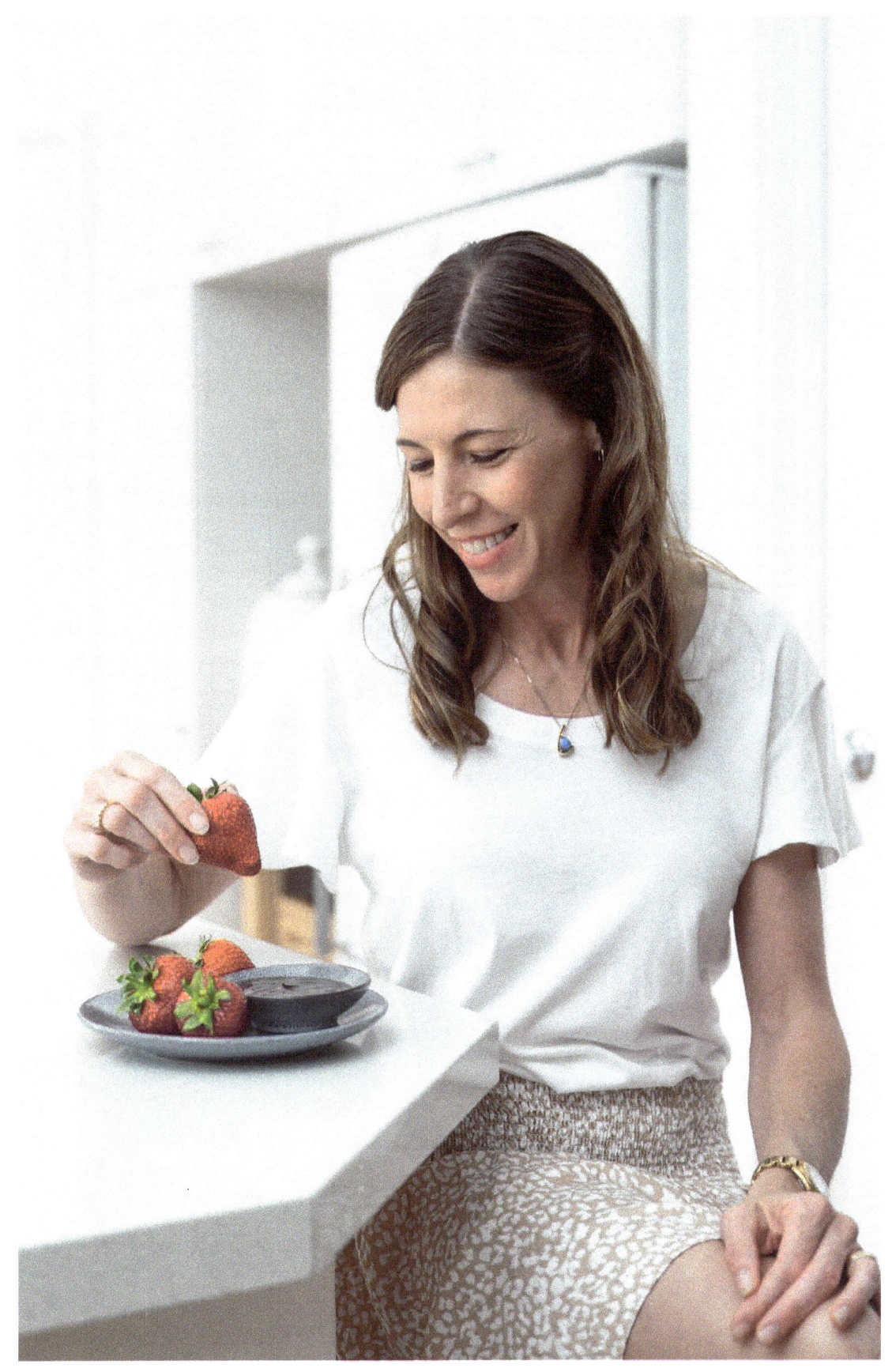

CONDIMENTS

CONDIMENTS

CASHEW NUT BUTTER

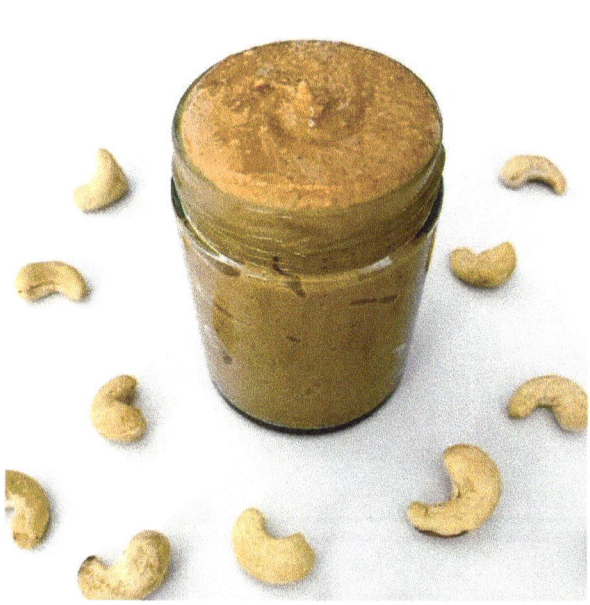

Prep. Time:	Make Time:	Makes:
10 min	6 min	220g

DIRECTIONS

1. Line a baking tray with baking paper. Spread the cashews evenly onto the tray.
2. Bake in the oven at 180°C for 10 MIN.
3. Allow to cool for 5 MIN.

Traditional ~ Place the cooled roasted cashews into a food processor and blend until the nut crumbs turn into a paste. Keep blending until you have a smooth creamy paste. This may take up to 5 MIN.

Add the oil and salt and blend again for 1 MIN.

Thermomix ~ Place the cooled roasted cashews into the TM bowl and blitz for 10 SEC / SP 10.

Then mix for 3 MIN / SP 4 to give you a smooth creamy paste.

Add the oil and salt. Mix for 30 SEC / SP 4.

~ ~ ~ ~ ~ ~ ~ ~ ~ ~ ~ ~ ~ ~ ~

Pour the nut butter into a sealable clean glass jar.

NOTES

Store in the pantry for up to 3 weeks.

You can use this as an alternative to peanut butter. Cashew butter is full of healthy fats and is high in protein and magnesium.

INGREDIENTS

- 270g (2 cups) Unsalted Cashews
- 15g (1 Tbsp) Cold Pressed Macadamia Nut Oil or Olive Oil
- Pinch of fine Sea Salt (optional)

CONDIMENTS

RASPBERRY CHIA JAM

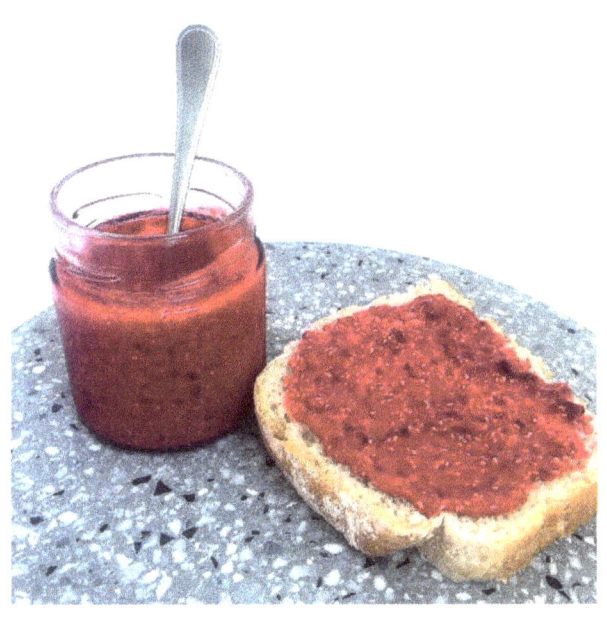

INGREDIENTS

- 45g (3 pitted) fresh Medjool Dates
- 100g (1 cup) Organic Frozen Raspberries
- 5g (1 tsp) Chia Seeds
- 10g (2 tsp) fresh Lemon Juice
- 20g (1 Tbsp) Pure Maple Syrup

Prep. Time:	Make Time:	Makes:
5 min	2 min	165g

DIRECTIONS

Traditional ~ Add the dates into a food processor and blitz together.

Scrape down the sides of the processing bowl and add the remaining ingredients. Blitz together for 1-2 MIN or until combined.

Thermomix ~ Add the dates into the TM bowl and blitz for 9 SEC / SP 9.

Scrape down the sides of the bowl and add the remaining ingredients. Blitz for 10 SEC / SP 10.

~ ~ ~ ~ ~ ~ ~ ~ ~ ~ ~ ~ ~ ~ ~

Pour the jam into a sealable clean glass jar. The mixture will look thick because of the frozen berries, however, once stored in the fridge, the berries will defrost and the jam will turn into a lovely consistency.

NOTES

Store the jam in the fridge for up to 2 weeks.

CONDIMENTS

CASHEW PARMESAN

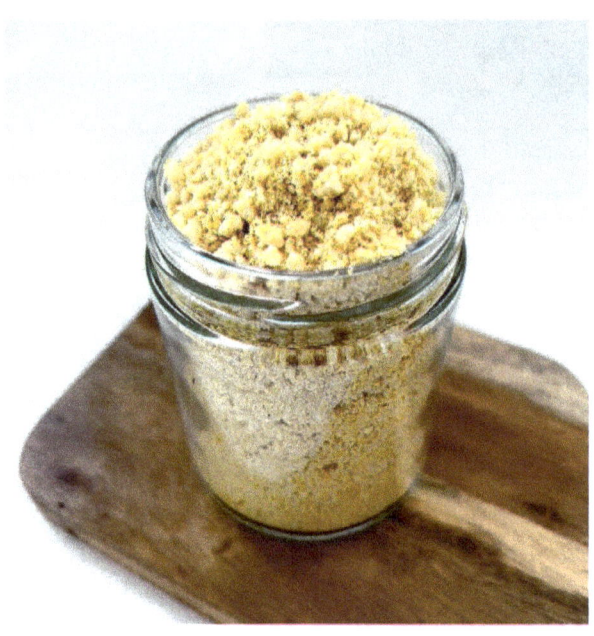

Prep. Time:	Make Time:	Makes:
2 min	1 min	150g

DIRECTIONS

Traditional ~ Add all the ingredients into a food processor and chop until a crumb consistency is achieved.

Thermomix ~ Add all the ingredients into the TM bowl and chop for 10 SEC / SP 5.

~ ~ ~ ~ ~ ~ ~ ~ ~ ~ ~ ~ ~ ~ ~

Pour the cashew parmesan into a sealable clean glass jar.

INGREDIENTS

- 1 cup (140g) Unsalted Cashews
- ¼ cup (20g) Nutritional Yeast
- ½ tsp fine Sea Salt
- ¾ tsp Garlic Powder

NOTES

Store in the freezer. It lasts for several weeks.

CONDIMENTS

VEGETABLE STOCK PASTE

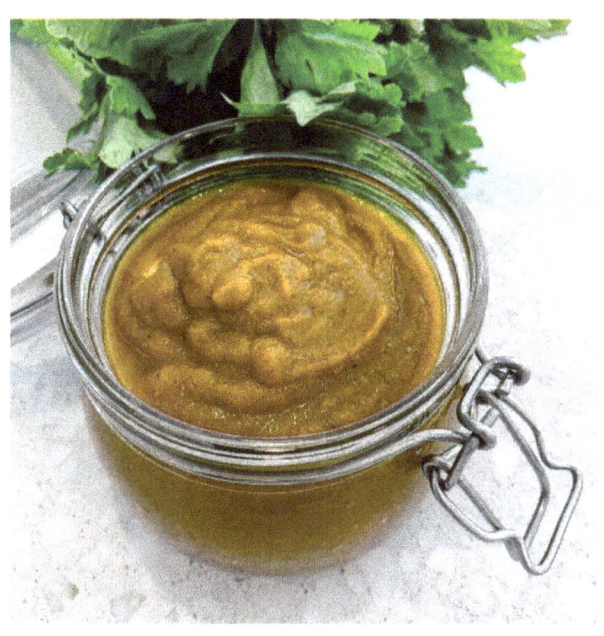

Prep. Time: 10 min
Cook Time: 15 min
Makes: 500g

DIRECTIONS

Traditional ~ Peel the onion, garlic and carrot. Finely dice all the vegetables and herbs, then place into a large saucepan. Add the salt and olive oil. Cook over a medium–low heat (with lid on) for 12-15 MIN, stirring frequently.

Once cooked, carefully use a stick mixer to blend until a paste forms.

Thermomix ~ Peel the onion, garlic and carrot. Roughly chop all the vegetables and herbs. Place these into the TM bowl and chop for 6 SEC / SP 5. Scrape down the sides of the bowl. Add the salt and olive oil. Cook for 14 MIN / 100°C / SP 1.

Blend together for 30 SEC starting on SP 5, working your way up to SP 9.

~ ~ ~ ~ ~ ~ ~ ~ ~ ~ ~ ~ ~ ~ ~

Empty the vegetable stock paste into a sealable clean glass jar and allow to cool before storing.

NOTES

Store in the fridge for up to 3 months.

1 Tbsp of vegetable stock paste is roughly equivalent to 1 stock cube.

INGREDIENTS

- 80g (2 sticks) Celery
- 100g (1 medium) Carrot
- 75g (½) Brown Onion
- 60g (½) Roma Tomato
- 140g (½) Zucchini
- 40g (2) Button Mushrooms
- ¼ small Capsicum
- 2 florets Broccoli
- 2 Garlic Cloves
- 1 sprig of Rosemary leaves
- 1 sprig of Parsley leaves
- 80g (¼ cup) Rock Salt
- 5g (1 tsp) Olive Oil

CONDIMENTS

CASHEW SOUR CREAM

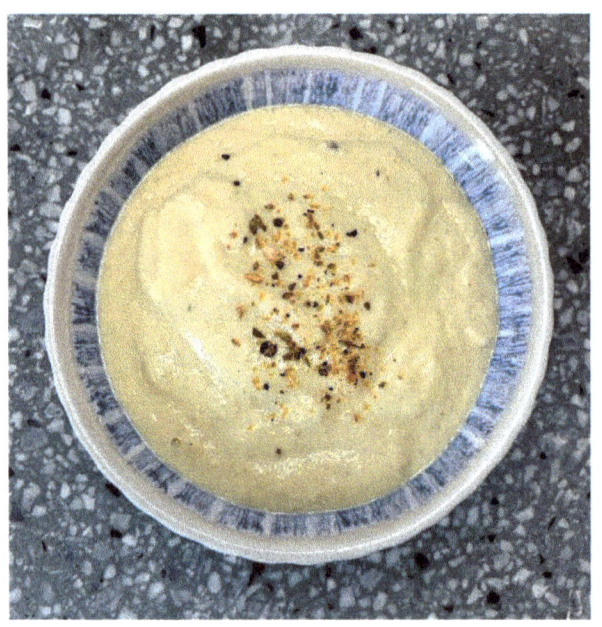

Prep. Time: 5 min
Make Time: 1 min
Makes: 215g

DIRECTIONS

Traditional ~ Add all the ingredients into a food processor and blend together until a creamy mixture forms.

Thermomix ~ Add all the ingredients into the TM bowl and blitz for 20 SEC / SP 10.

~ ~ ~ ~ ~ ~ ~ ~ ~ ~ ~ ~ ~ ~ ~

Empty the cream mixture into a small bowl and serve immediately.

INGREDIENTS

- 140g (1 cup) Unsalted Cashews
- 125g (½ cup) Filtered Water
- 15g (1 Tbsp) fresh Lemon Juice
- 5g (1 tsp) Organic Apple Cider Vinegar
- 2 tsp Nutritional Yeast Flakes
- ½ tsp fine Sea Salt

NOTES

Store any leftovers in an airtight container in the fridge for up to 4 days. It does begin to thicken up in the fridge, so if you like it a little runnier use it straight away.

This is a great topping for the Nacho's recipe (pg. 92).

CONDIMENTS

CASHEW AIOLI

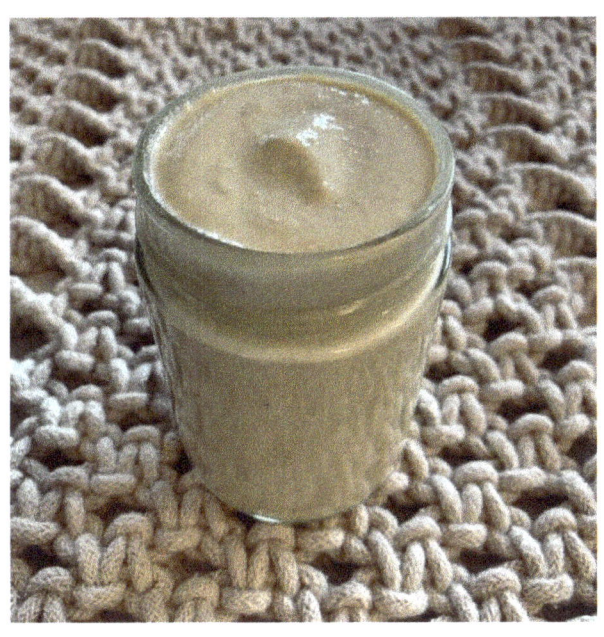

Prep. Time: 15 min | Make Time: 3 min | Makes: 300g

DIRECTIONS

1. Place the cashews into a heat proof bowl. Cover the nuts with the boiling water, place a lid on top and set aside for 10-15 MIN.
2. Drain off the excess liquid.

Traditional ~ Place the drained nuts into a blender with the mustard, lemon juice, peeled garlic, apple cider vinegar, salt and coconut sugar. Blend on high for 1 MIN or until you have a chunky paste. Scrape down the sides of the blender. With the motor running on low, slowly drizzle the macadamia oil in. Add the water and blitz on high again for 2 MIN or until the aioli is smooth.

Thermomix ~ Place the drained nuts into the TM bowl with the mustard, lemon juice, peeled garlic, apple cider vinegar, salt and coconut sugar. Blitz for 5 SEC / SP 9.

Scrape down the sides of the bowl. Turn the speed to 3, then pour the oil onto the TM lid, so it slowly drips through and under the MC (measuring cup). This should take 1 MIN. Scrape down the sides of the bowl, then add the water and blitz on high again for 10 SEC / SP 10.

~~~~~~~~~~~~~~~

Place the aioli into a dipping bowl for serving.

INGREDIENTS

- 140g (1 cup) Unsalted Cashews
- 40g (2 Tbsp + 2 tsp) Dijon Mustard
- 30g (2 Tbsp) fresh Lemon Juice
- 1 Garlic Clove
- 20g (1 Tbsp +1 tsp) Organic Apple Cider Vinegar
- ½ tsp fine Sea Salt
- 5g (1 tsp) Coconut Sugar
- 110g (½ cup) Macadamia Oil (or Olive Oil)
- 85g (⅓ cup) Filtered Water

NOTES

Store any leftovers in an airtight container in the fridge for up to 4 days.

This is an amazing dipping sauce for the baked seasoned wedges (pg. 106).

CONDIMENTS

CREAMY DILL DRESSING

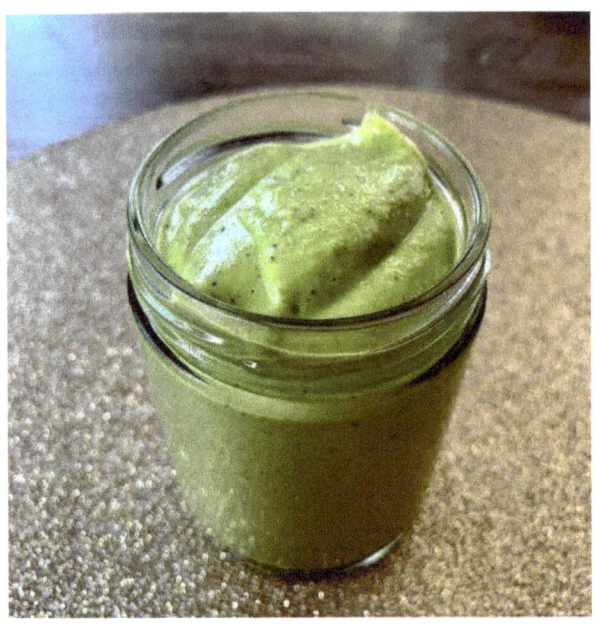

Prep. Time:	Make Time:	Makes:
15 min	3 min	420g

DIRECTIONS

1. Place the cashews into a heat proof bowl. Cover the nuts with the boiling water, place a lid on top and set aside for 10-15 MIN.
2. Drain off the excess liquid.

Traditional ~ Place the drained nuts into a food processor along with all the remaining ingredients. Blitz together until smooth.

Thermomix ~ Place the drained nuts into the TM bowl along with all the remaining ingredients. Blitz together for 10 SEC / SP 10.

~ ~ ~ ~ ~ ~ ~ ~ ~ ~ ~ ~ ~ ~ ~

Serve over salads or cooked vegetables.

NOTES

Store any leftovers in an airtight container in the fridge for up to 4 days.

INGREDIENTS

- 150g (1 cup) Unsalted Cashews
- 10g (¼ cup) Fresh Dill
- 50g (2 Tbsp) Organic Apple Cider Vinegar
- 40g (2 Tbsp) Pure Maple Syrup
- 40g (2 Tbsp) Dijon Mustard
- 1 Garlic Clove (peeled)
- Squeeze of fresh Lemon Juice
- 125g (½ cup) Almond Milk
- Pinch of fine Sea Salt

CONDIMENTS

MEXICAN SPICE MIX

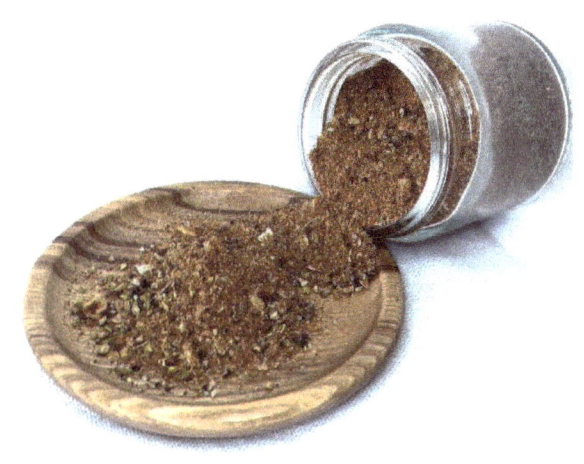

Prep. Time:	Make Time:	Makes:
2 min	1 min	60g

DIRECTIONS

Traditional ~ Place all the ingredients into a bowl and stir to combine.

Thermomix ~ Place all the ingredients into the TM bowl and mix for 10 SEC / SP 3.

~ ~ ~ ~ ~ ~ ~ ~ ~ ~ ~ ~ ~ ~ ~

Pour the spice mix into a sealable clean glass jar.

NOTES

Store in the pantry for up to 3 months.

INGREDIENTS

- 10g (4 tsp) ground Cumin
- 10g (4 tsp) ground Black Pepper
- 10g (4 tsp) fine Sea Salt
- 5g (2 tsp) dried Oregano
- 5g (2 tsp) ground Paprika
- 1 tsp Garlic Powder
- 1 tsp Onion Powder

CONDIMENTS

TUSCAN SEASONING MIX

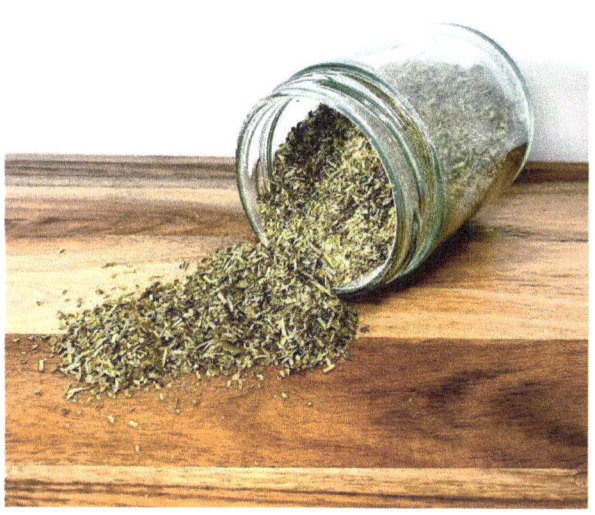

INGREDIENTS

- 10g (4 tsp) dried Rosemary
- 10g (4 tsp) dried Oregano
- 10g (4 tsp) dried Basil
- 15g (4 tsp) Garlic Powder
- 5g (1 tsp) fine Sea Salt
- 5g (1 tsp) ground Black Pepper

Prep. Time:	Make Time:	Makes:
2 min	1 min	20g

DIRECTIONS

Traditional ~ Place all the ingredients into a bowl and stir to combine.

Thermomix ~ Place all the ingredients into the TM bowl and mix for 10 SEC / SP 3.

~ ~ ~ ~ ~ ~ ~ ~ ~ ~ ~ ~ ~ ~ ~

Pour the seasoning mix into a sealable clean glass jar.

NOTES

Store in the pantry for up to 3 months.

CONDIMENTS

CHOCOLATE DRINKING POWDER

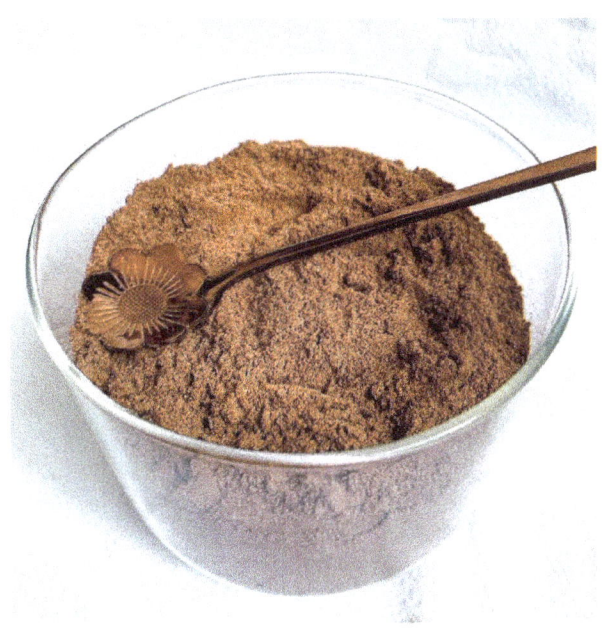

Prep. Time:	Make Time:	Makes:
5 min	2 min	200g

DIRECTIONS

Traditional ~ Add the sunflower kernels, pepita seeds, vanilla and sugar to a food processor and blitz until you have a fine crumb. Add the cacao powder and mix until combined.

Thermomix ~ Add the sunflower kernels, pepita seeds, vanilla and sugar to the TM bowl and blitz for 10 SEC / SP 10. Add the cacao powder and mix for 10 SEC / SP 4.

~~~~~~~~~~~~~~~

Pour into a sealable clean glass jar.

NOTES

Store for up to 3 months in the pantry.

Use 2 Tbsp of chocolate powder with 1 cup of warm or cold plant-based milk of your choice. Whisk to combine and enjoy.

This is a hot chocolate like no other, as it is full of vitamins and minerals which support the immune system.

INGREDIENTS

- 20g (2 Tbsp) Sunflower Kernels
- 20g (2 Tbsp) Pepita Seeds
- 1 Vanilla Bean (whole and cut into 4 pieces) OR ¼ tsp Vanilla Bean Powder
- 110g (½ cup) Organic Raw Sugar
- 50g (½ cup) Organic Cacao Powder

CONDIMENTS

CHOCOLATE DIPPING SAUCE

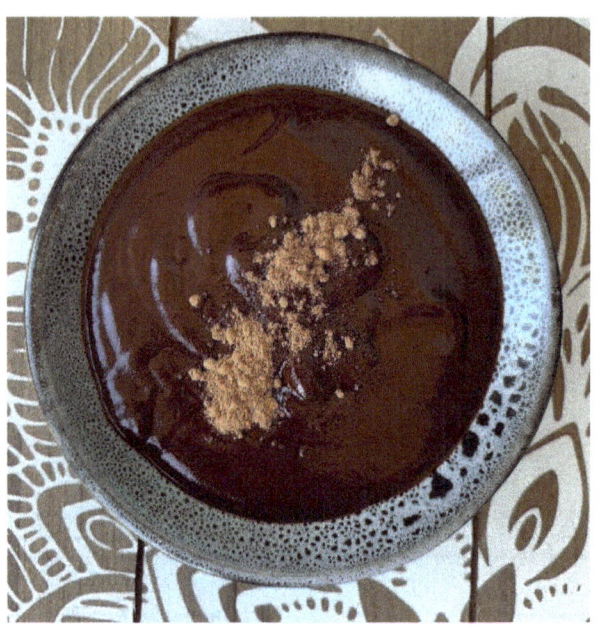

Prep. Time:	Make Time:	Makes:
2 min	2 min	70g

DIRECTIONS

Traditional ~ Melt the coconut oil in a small heat proof bowl in the microwave for 30 SEC. Add the remaining ingredients and whisk together until smooth.

Thermomix ~ Add the coconut oil to the TM bowl and melt for 1 MIN / 37°C / SP STIR.

Add the remaining ingredients to the TM bowl and mix for 6 SEC / SP 4.

~ ~ ~ ~ ~ ~ ~ ~ ~ ~ ~ ~ ~ ~ ~

Pour into a small bowl and serve. Dip fresh fruit like strawberries or bananas, or drizzle over waffles, pancakes or dairy free ice-cream.

INGREDIENTS

- 30g (2 Tbsp) Organic Coconut Oil
- 20g (1 Tbsp) Pure Maple Syrup
- 15g (3 Tbsp) Organic Cacao Powder
- Pinch of fine Sea Salt

NOTES

Add a drop of food grade peppermint or orange essential oil for a lovely flavour.

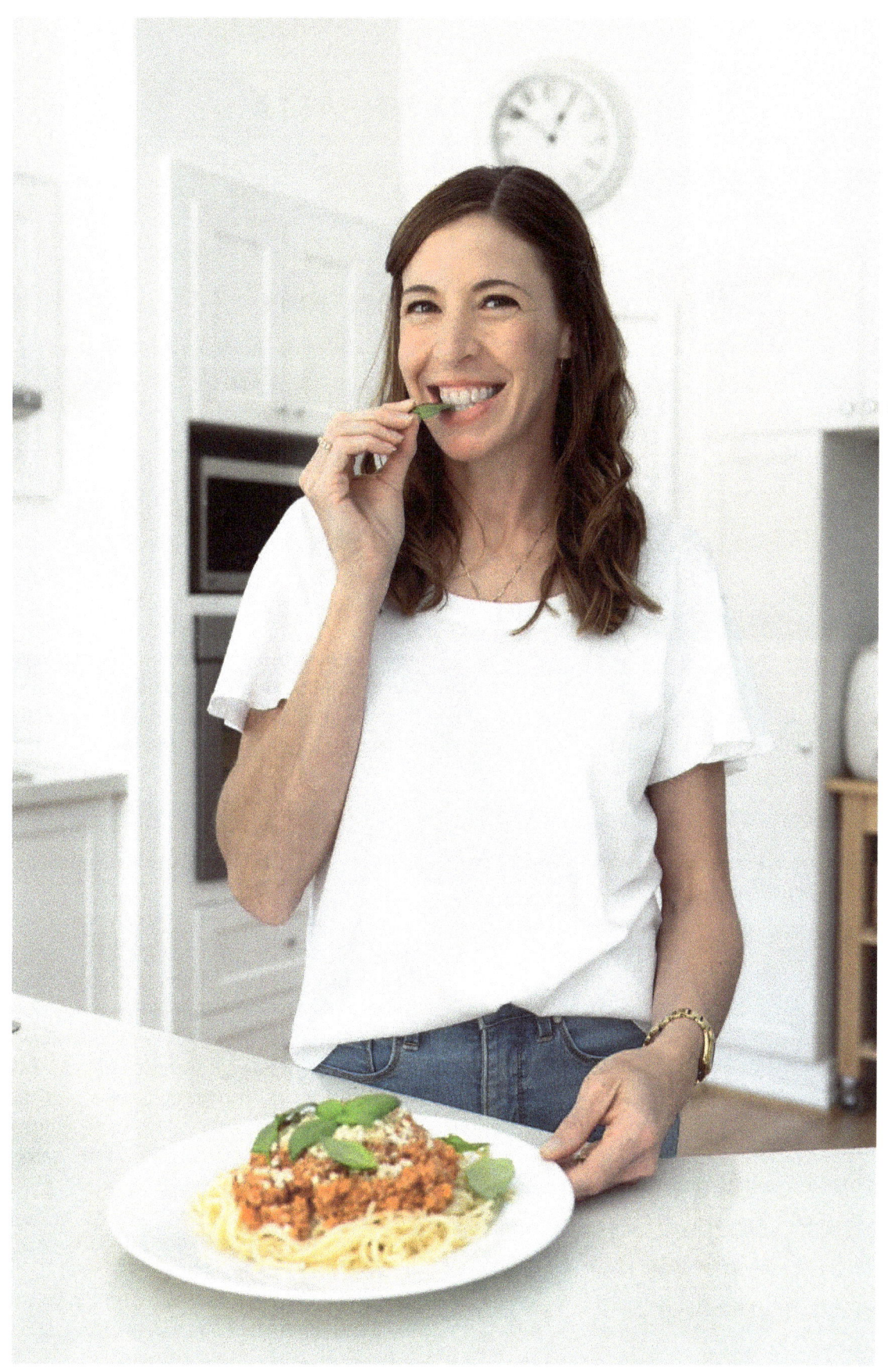

DINNERS

DINNER

CREAMY TOMATO PASTA

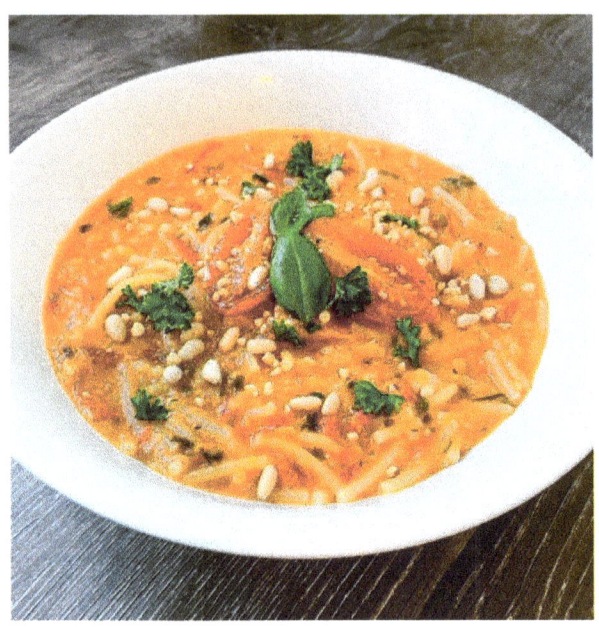

Prep. Time:	Cook Time:	Serves:
10 min	25 min	4

DIRECTIONS

1. Prepare the cashew parmesan (pg. 64) and set aside.

Traditional ~ Peel the onion and garlic. Finely dice the onion, garlic, 5 sprigs of parsley leaves, capsicum, zucchini and mushroom. Add these to a large saucepan with the olive oil. Sauté over a medium heat (with the lid on) for 5 MIN, stirring regularly.

Add the quartered tomatoes, water, vegetable stock paste, coconut cream and cashew parmesan to the saucepan. Cook (with the lid on) for 10 MIN over a medium heat, stirring regularly.

Snap the pasta into halves and submerge in the sauce. Cook for another 10 MIN over a medium-low heat (with the lid on), stirring regularly.

~ ~ ~ ~ ~ ~ ~ ~ ~ ~ ~ ~ ~ ~

Thermomix ~ Peel the onion and garlic. Place the onion, garlic and 5 sprigs of parsley leaves into the TM and chop for 3 SEC / SP 7. Scrape down the sides of the TM bowl. Roughly chop the capsicum, zucchini, and mushroom and place into the TM bowl. Chop for 3 SEC / SP 5 then scrape down the sides of the bowl. Add the olive oil and sauté for 3 MIN / VAROMA / SP 1.

Add the quartered tomatoes, water, vegetable stock paste, coconut cream and cashew parmesan. Cook for 10 MIN / 100°C / SP 1. Snap the pasta into halves and submerge in the sauce. Cook for 10 MIN / 100°C / SP STIR.

~ ~ ~ ~ ~ ~ ~ ~ ~ ~ ~ ~ ~ ~

Serve and garnish with fresh parsley and sprinkle with the cashew parmesan.

INGREDIENTS

- 75g (½ medium) Brown Onion
- 2 Garlic Cloves
- 6 sprigs of fresh Parsley (leaves only – keep 1 sprig aside for serving)
- 250g (1 medium) Red Capsicum
- 140g (½) Zucchini
- 60g (1) Portobello Mushroom
- 575g (5) Roma Tomatoes
- 30g (2 Tbsp) Olive Oil
- 375g (1 ½ cups) Filtered Water
- 20g (1 Tbsp) Vegetable Stock Paste (pg. 65)
- 180g (¾ cup + 1 Tbsp) Organic Coconut Cream
- 40g (⅓ cup) Cashew Parmesan (pg. 64)
- 250g Fettuccini or Spaghetti

SERVING INGREDIENTS

- Cashew Parmesan
- Parsley leaves

DINNER

STUFFED MUSHROOMS

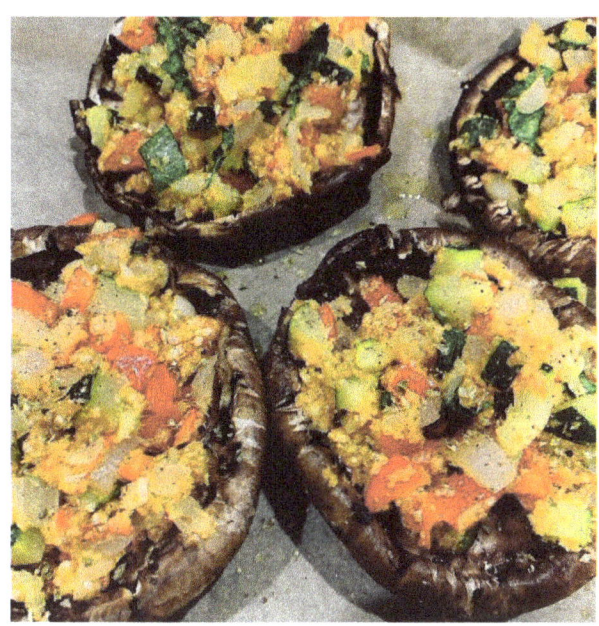

INGREDIENTS

- 240g (4) Portobello Mushrooms
- 2 Garlic Cloves
- 75g (½ medium) Brown Onion
- 140g (½) Zucchini
- 125g (½ medium) Capsicum
- 115g (1) Roma Tomato
- 25g (¼ cup) Breadcrumbs
- 40g (¼ cup) Cashew Parmesan (pg. 64)
- Pinch of dried Coriander
- Pinch of dried Oregano
- Pinch of fine Sea Salt
- Pinch of ground Black Pepper
- 30g (2 Tbsp) Olive Oil

Prep. Time:	Cook Time:	Serves:
10 min	35 min	4

DIRECTIONS – Traditional Only

1. Wash and pat dry the mushrooms, then scrape the gills out with a spoon and cut the stalks off.

2. Line a baking tray with baking paper, then place the mushrooms hollowed side facing up. Drizzle with olive oil and set aside.

Traditional ~ Peel the onion and garlic. Finely dice the onion, garlic, zucchini, capsicum and tomato. Place these into a large frypan with 1 Tbsp olive oil. Sauté for 2 MIN over a medium heat.

Add the remaining ingredients and continue to cook for 8 MIN stirring frequently.

Thermomix ~ Peel the onion and garlic and place into the TM bowl. Roughly chop the zucchini, capsicum and tomato and add into the TM bowl. Chop for 3 SEC / SP 4. Add 1 Tbsp olive oil and sauté for 3 MIN / VAROMA / SP 1.

Add the remaining ingredients and cook for 6 MIN / 100˚C / SP STIR.

~ ~ ~ ~ ~ ~ ~ ~ ~ ~ ~ ~ ~ ~

Scoop the vegetable mixture evenly into the oiled mushrooms.

Bake in the oven at 180°C for 25 MIN.

Serve on plates and enjoy.

DINNER

VEGETABLE PIE

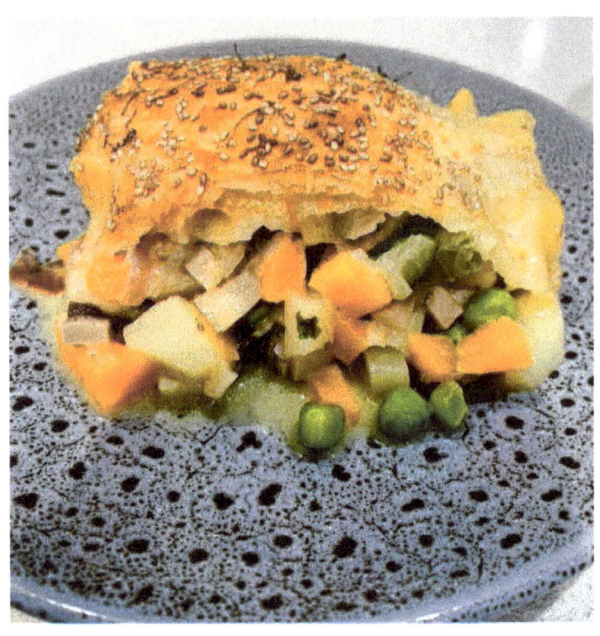

Prep. Time: 10 min
Cook Time: 45 min
Serves: 4

INGREDIENTS

- 15g (1 Tbsp) Olive Oil
- 2 Garlic Cloves
- 70g (½ medium) Red Onion
- 45g (1 stick) Celery
- 200g (2 medium) Carrots
- 160g (½) Zucchini
- 220g (1 medium) Potato
- 60g (1) Portobello Mushroom
- 40g (⅓ cup) Frozen Peas
- 190g (¾ cup) Organic Coconut Cream
- 20g (1 Tbsp) Vegetable Stock Paste (pg. 65)
- 5g (1 Tbsp) Nutritional Yeast
- ¼ tsp ground Black Pepper
- 2 Tbsp fresh Coriander leaves
- ½ tsp Dijon Mustard
- Handful of Spinach Leaves
- 1 sheet of dairy free Puff Pastry
- 1-2 tsp Chia Seeds
- Splash of Almond Milk or Coconut Cream

DIRECTIONS

Traditional ~ Peel and finely dice the onion and garlic. Thinly slice the celery. Add the oil to a large frypan and sauté the garlic, onion and celery together. Peel and dice the carrot and potato into 1cm cubes. Dice the zucchini. Add these vegetables to the frypan. Cook for 5 MIN, over a medium heat with the lid on, stirring occasionally.

Dice the mushrooms and add to the frypan along with the peas, coconut cream, vegetable stock paste, nutritional yeast, pepper, coriander and mustard. Simmer with the lid on for 10 MIN. Turn off the heat and stir through the spinach leaves. Empty the pie filling into a large pie dish.

Thermomix ~ Peel the onion and garlic, roughly chop the celery and add these into the TM bowl. Chop for 5 SEC / SP 4. Scrape down the sides of the bowl and add the oil. Sauté for 3 MIN / VAROMA / SP STIR.

Roughly cut the zucchini, carrots, potato and mushroom. Add these into the TM bowl and chop for 10 SEC / SP 4. Scrape down the sides of the bowl. Cook for 5 MIN / 100°C / REVERSE / SP 1.

Add the remaining ingredients (except the spinach leaves) to the TM bowl. Cook for 10 MIN / 100°C / REVERSE / SP 1. Add the spinach leaves and stir for 5 SEC / REVERSE / SP 2. Empty the pie filling into a large pie dish.

~ ~ ~ ~ ~ ~ ~ ~ ~ ~ ~ ~ ~ ~ ~

Press the defrosted puff pastry into the edges of the dish. Brush the pastry with some of the excess coconut cream or a little almond milk and sprinkle the chia seeds over the top.

Bake in the oven at 200°C for 30 MIN.

Cut into quarters and serve on plates.

DINNER

QUINOA BOLOGNESE

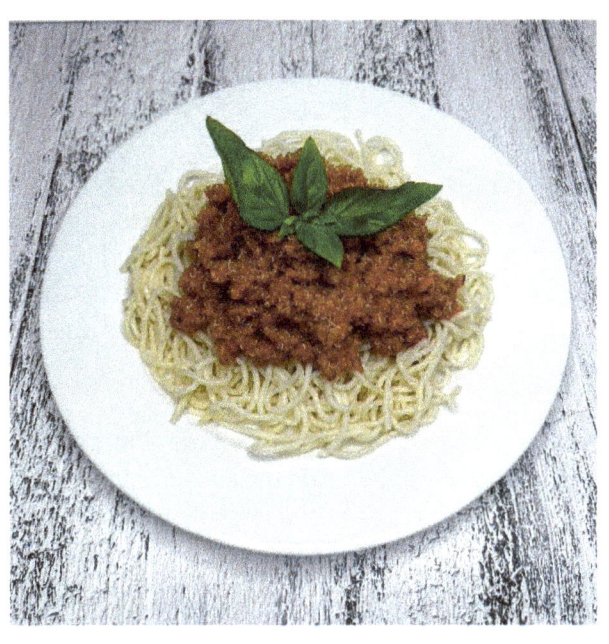

Prep. Time: 10 min   **Cook Time:** 13 min   **Serves:** 4

DIRECTIONS

1. Rinse the quinoa under water using a sieve. Add the quinoa to a small saucepan with the water. Bring to a boil, then turn the heat to simmer and cook until the water is absorbed.

2. In a medium size saucepan, bring 2L of water with a pinch of salt to the boil. Add the spaghetti and cook until al dente.

Traditional ~ Peel and finely dice the onion and garlic. Peel and grate the carrots. Finely slice the celery. Add these to a large frypan with the olive oil. Sauté over a low heat for 5 MIN.

Add the jar of passata sauce, vegetable stock paste, nutritional yeast, tamari sauce and seasoning. Stir together for 5 MIN. Add the cooked quinoa to the frypan and stir together for 2 MIN.

Thermomix ~ See pg. 5 for the TM way to cook quinoa. Using the TM to cook the quinoa will just increase the overall cooking time.

Peel and place the onion and garlic into the TM bowl and chop for 1 SEC / SP 7. Scrape down the sides of the bowl. Add the olive oil. Sauté for 3 MIN / VAROMA / SP 1.

Wash and roughly chop the carrot and celery. Add into the TM bowl. Chop for 4 SEC / SP 6. Add the remaining ingredients. Cook for 9 MIN / 100°C / SP STIR. Add the cooked quinoa into the TM bowl and mix for 30 SEC / 100°C / SP 4.

~ ~ ~ ~ ~ ~ ~ ~ ~ ~ ~ ~ ~ ~ ~

Drain the cooked spaghetti. Serve in bowls with the quinoa bolognese. Add the cashew parmesan and fresh basil leaves on top.

INGREDIENTS

- 150g (¾ cup) Quinoa
- 250g (1 cup) Filtered Water
- 250g – 300g Spaghetti
- 75g (½ medium) Brown Onion
- 2 Garlic Cloves
- 200g (2 medium) Carrots
- 45g (1 stick) Celery
- 15g (1 Tbsp) Olive Oil
- 1 x 700g jar Passata
- 20g (1 Tbsp) Vegetable Stock Paste (pg. 65)
- 7g (2 Tbsp) Nutritional Yeast
- 5g (1 tsp) Organic Tamari Sauce
- 1 Tbsp Tuscan Seasoning (pg. 70)

SERVING INGREDIENTS

- Cashew Parmesan (pg. 64)
- Fresh Basil Leaves

DINNER

CURRIED COCONUT PUMPKIN SOUP

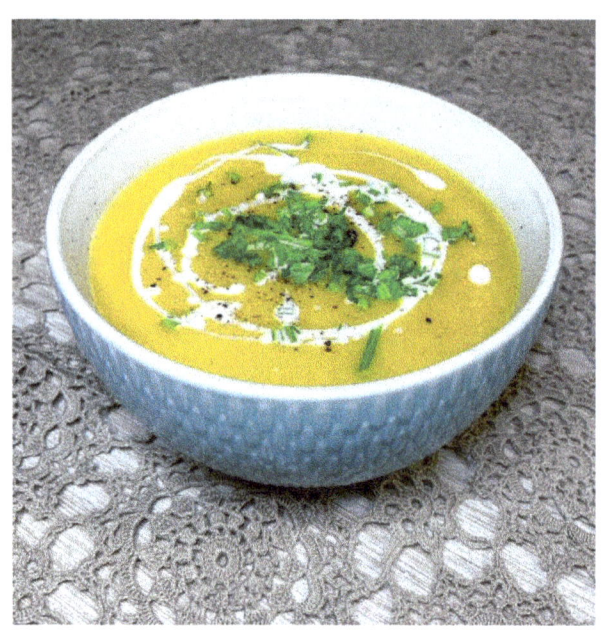

Prep. Time:	Cook Time:	Serves:
10 min	30 min	4

DIRECTIONS

Traditional ~ Peel and dice the onion and garlic and add to a large saucepan with the olive oil and curry powder. Sauté over a medium heat for 5 MIN.

Peel and cut the pumpkin, potato and sweet potato into 2cm cubes. Add the cubed vegetables, vegetable stock paste, coriander leaves, tamari sauce and water to the saucepan. Cover and bring to a boil, then reduce the heat and simmer for 25 MIN, stirring frequently.

Add the coconut cream. Using a stick mixer, blend the cooked vegetables and liquid together until you have a soup consistency. (If using a blender, use half the mixture at a time to prevent the hot liquid exploding everywhere).

Thermomix ~ Peel the onion and garlic. Add to the TM bowl and chop for 1 SEC / SP 7. Scrape down the sides of the bowl. Add the olive oil and curry powder. Sauté for 3 MIN / VAROMA / SP 1.

Peel and cut the pumpkin, potato and sweet potato into 2cm cubes. Add the cubed vegetables, vegetable stock paste, coriander leaves, tamari sauce and water to the TM bowl and cook for 25 MIN / 100°C / SP 1.

Slowly turn the speed dial up to SP 4 until the machine is balanced and no longer vibrates. Then, slowly turn the speed dial up to SP 9 (this should take 1 MIN). Add the coconut cream and mix for 5 SEC / SP 4.

~ ~ ~ ~ ~ ~ ~ ~ ~ ~ ~ ~ ~ ~

Serve in bowls and season with pepper, fresh coriander and a drizzle of coconut cream.

INGREDIENTS

- 75g (½ medium) Brown Onion
- 4 Garlic Cloves
- 5g (2 tsp) Indian Curry Powder
- 15g (1 Tbsp) Olive Oil
- 600g (½) Butternut Pumpkin
- 220g (1 medium) Potato
- 300g (¾ medium) Sweet Potato
- 40g (2 Tbsp) Vegetable Stock Paste (pg. 65)
- 1 Tbsp Fresh Coriander Leaves
- ½ tsp Organic Tamari Sauce
- 500g (2 cups) Filtered Water
- 180g (¾ cup) Organic Coconut Cream

SERVING INGREDIENTS

- Fresh Coriander Leaves
- Ground Black Pepper
- Organic Coconut Cream

DINNER

CHEESY BROCCOLI PASTA

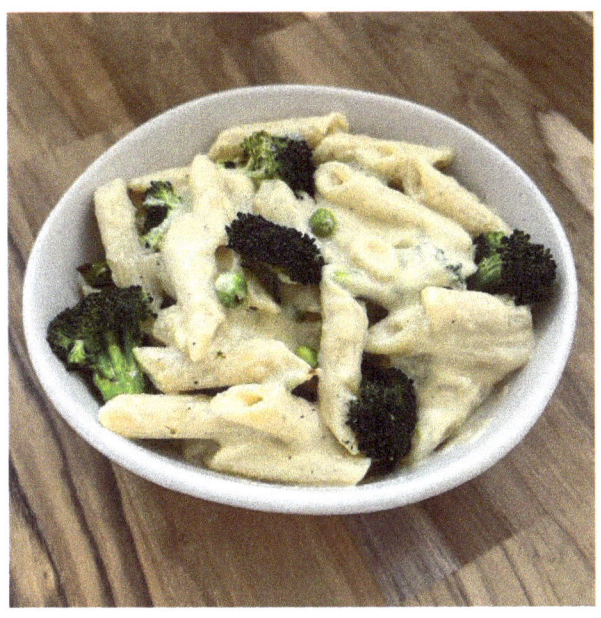

Prep. Time: 15 min
Cook Time: 30 min
Serves: 4

INGREDIENTS

- 300g (approx. 3 cups) Penne Pasta
- 200g (1 large) Brown Onion
- 15g (5) Garlic Cloves
- 375g (1 ½ cups) Filtered Water
- 10g (2 tsp) Vegetable Stock Paste (pg. 65)
- ½ tsp ground Black Pepper
- 150g (1 cup) Unsalted Cashews
- 15g (1 Tbsp) Lemon Juice
- 25g (¼ cup) Nutritional Yeast
- 5g (1 tsp) Dijon Mustard
- 40g (¼ cup) Frozen Peas
- ½ head of Broccoli

DIRECTIONS

1. Add the cashews to a heat proof dish and cover with boiling water. Allow this to sit for 10-15 MIN.
2. In a large pot, add 2L filtered water and a pinch of salt. Bring to the boil. Add the pasta and cook as per packet instructions.
3. Slice the broccoli into small pieces. Place on a baking tray with baking paper. Drizzle with olive oil. Season with salt and pepper. Bake in the oven at 180°C for 15 MIN.

Traditional ~ Peel and finely dice the onion and garlic. Add to a large saucepan with the vegetable stock paste and 1 cup of water. Stir and cook for 10 MIN or until the liquid reduces.

Add ½ cup water, pepper, lemon juice, nutritional yeast, mustard and drained cashews. Using a stick mixer, blend the sauce together.

Add the peas and cook for 5 MIN over a low heat, stirring regularly. Drain the cooked pasta. Add the pasta into the saucepan and stir together. Serve in bowls.

Thermomix ~ Peel the onion and garlic. Cut the onion in half. Add these into the TM bowl and chop for 2 SEC / SP 7.

Add the vegetable stock paste and 250g of water. Cook for 10 MIN / 100°C / SP STIR.

Add 125g water, pepper, lemon juice, nutritional yeast, mustard and the drained cashews. Blitz for 1 MIN / SP 9.

Add the peas and cook for 5 MIN / 100°C / REVERSE / SP STIR. Drain the cooked pasta. Add the pasta and broccoli into the TM bowl. Mix for 10 SEC / REVERSE / SP 3. Serve in bowls.

DINNER

JACKFRUIT TACOS

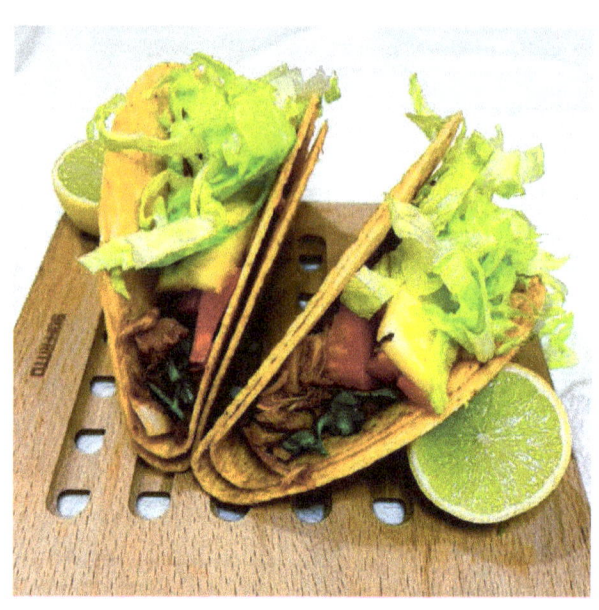

Prep. Time:	Cook Time:	Serves:
10 min	15 min	4

DIRECTIONS

1. Line a baking tray with baking paper. Place the taco shells on the tray and bake in the oven at 180°C for 5-10 MIN.

Traditional ~ Rinse and thoroughly pat dry the jackfruit, then shred it into small pieces and set aside. Peel and dice the onion and garlic. In a large frypan, add the onion, garlic and olive oil. Sauté over a low heat for 2 MIN. Then add the shredded jackfruit and all remaining ingredients. Simmer over a low heat for 5-10 MIN, stirring occasionally.

Thermomix ~ Peel the onion and garlic and place into the TM bowl. Chop for 1 SEC / SP 7. Scrape down the sides of the bowl. Add the oil and sauté for 3 MIN / VAROMA / SP 1. Rinse and thoroughly pat dry the jackfruit. Add the jackfruit into the TM bowl and chop for 4 SEC / SP 4. Scrape down the sides of the bowl. Add all remaining ingredients. Cook for 5 MIN / 100°C / REVERSE / SP STIR.

~ ~ ~ ~ ~ ~ ~ ~ ~ ~ ~ ~ ~ ~ ~

Prepare the additional serving ingredients for the tacos.

Remove the taco shells from the oven. Scoop a small amount of the jackfruit mixture into each taco shell, then layer the serving ingredients on top.

Serve on plates and enjoy.

INGREDIENTS

- 1 x 400g tin Organic Jackfruit
- 70g (½ medium) Red Onion
- 2 Garlic Cloves
- 15g (1 Tbsp) Olive Oil
- 10g (2 tsp) ground Cumin
- 5g (2 tsp) ground Paprika
- 5g (3 tsp) Mexican Spice Mix (pg. 69)
- 10g (2 tsp) Sweet Chilli Sauce
- 20g (1 Tbsp) Pure Maple Syrup
- 20g (1 Tbsp) Vegetable Stock Paste (pg. 65)
- 45g (3 Tbsp) Filtered Water
- 5g (2 Tbsp) Fresh Coriander Leaves (sliced) / 1 tsp dried coriander
- Juice of 1 fresh Lime
- 1 x 10 - 12 packet of Taco Shells

SERVING INGREDIENTS

- 1 Tomato (diced)
- 2 Pineapple rings (sliced)
- sliced cos lettuce or spinach leaves.

DINNER

ZUCCHINI CAULIFLOWER CORN SOUP

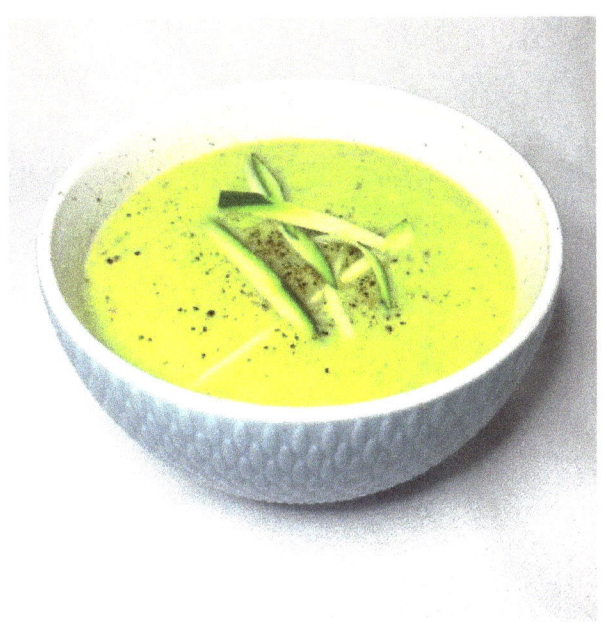

Prep. Time: 5 min   Cook Time: 25 min   Serves: 4

DIRECTIONS

Traditional ~ Peel and finely dice the onion and garlic. Place these into a medium saucepan with the olive oil and sauté for 5 MIN, stirring frequently. Quarter then roughly cut the zucchini. Slice the cauliflower florets into halves. Drain and rinse the corn kernels. Add these vegetables, plus the water and vegetable stock paste to the saucepan. Over a medium–low heat, with the lid on, cook for 20 MIN, stirring frequently.

Using a stick mixer, blend until you have a soup consistency.

Thermomix ~ Peel and place the onion and garlic into the TM bowl and chop for 1 SEC / SP 7. Scrape down the sides of the bowl and add the olive oil. Sauté for 3 MIN / VAROMA / SP 1.

Add the water and vegetable stock paste into the TM bowl. Roughly chop the zucchini and cauliflower. Place these into the simmering basket along with the drained corn kernels (the simmering basket should be filled to the top). Insert the simmering basket into the TM bowl. Cook for 20 MIN / VAROMA / SP 3.

Empty the basket of cooked vegetables into the liquid mixture in the TM bowl. Blend for 1 MIN, gradually increasing the speed from SP 1 – SP 9.

~ ~ ~ ~ ~ ~ ~ ~ ~ ~ ~ ~ ~ ~ ~

Serve in bowls. Add some ground black pepper and thinly sliced zucchini on top. This is also delicious with some additive free fresh bread.

INGREDIENTS

- 150g (1 medium) Brown Onion
- 2 Garlic Cloves
- 15g (1 Tbsp) Olive Oil
- 20g (1 Tbsp) Vegetable Stock Paste (pg. 65)
- 500g (2 cups) Filtered Water
- 160g (½) Zucchini
- 360g (½) Cauliflower
- 125g (½ cup) Corn Kernels

SERVING INGREDIENTS

- Ground Black Pepper
- Zucchini (thinly sliced)
- Fresh Bread

DINNER

TUSCAN QUINOA BALLS

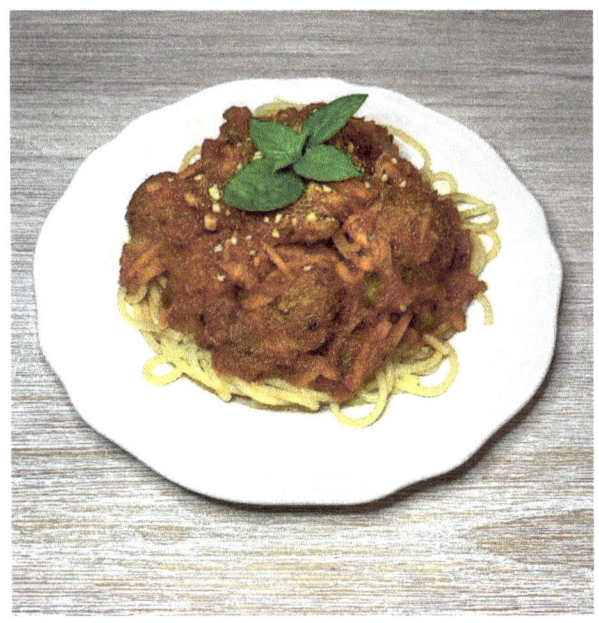

INGREDIENTS

TUSCAN QUINOA BALLS

- 200g (1 cup) Quinoa
- 360g (1 ½ cups) Filtered Water / 1000g Filtered Water for TM
- 5g (1 Tbsp) Tuscan Seasoning Mix (pg. 70)
- 25g (⅓ cup) Breadcrumbs
- 10g (2 Tbsp) Nutritional Yeast
- 40g (2 Tbsp) Tomato Paste
- 20g (1 Tbsp) Vegetable Stock Paste (pg. 65)
- 5g (1 tsp) Organic Tamari Sauce
- 2g (1 tsp) ground Paprika
- 40g (¼ cup) Coconut Flour

TUSCAN SAUCE

- 75g (½ medium) Brown Onion
- 3 Garlic Cloves
- 45g (1 stick) Celery
- 100g (1 medium) Carrot
- 15g (1 Tbsp) Olive Oil
- 2 x 400g tinned Diced Tomatoes
- 40g (2 Tbsp) Tomato Paste
- 5g (1 Tbsp) Tuscan Seasoning Mix (pg. 70)
- 5g (1 tsp) Organic Tamari Sauce
- 65g (¼ cup) Filtered Water

SERVING

- 250g Spaghetti
- Fresh Basil Leaves
- Cashew Parmesan (pg. 64)

DINNER

TUSCAN QUINOA BALLS (CONTINUED)

Prep. Time: 12 min
Cook Time: 55 min
Serves: 4

DIRECTIONS

TUSCAN QUINOA BALLS

Traditional ~ Add 1 cup quinoa with 1 ½ cups filtered water to a small saucepan with a lid. Bring to a boil over a medium heat, then reduce the heat to a simmer. Cook for 10 MIN or until all the liquid is absorbed.

Meanwhile, add the remaining quinoa ball ingredients to a large bowl. Allow the cooked quinoa to cool slightly, before adding it into the bowl. Stir together until combined.

Thermomix ~ Insert the TM simmering basket into the TM bowl. Pour in the 1000g filtered water, then place the quinoa into the simmering basket. Cook for 15 MIN / 100°C / SP 4.

Once the quinoa has cooked, remove the simmering basket and discard the liquid. Return the cooked quinoa into the TM bowl and add the remaining quinoa ball ingredients. Mix for 30 SEC / REVERSE / SP 3.

~ ~ ~ ~ ~ ~ ~ ~ ~ ~ ~ ~ ~ ~ ~

Using slightly wet hands, scoop tablespoon amounts of quinoa mixture in the palms of your hands and roll into balls. This should make 22 balls.

Line a baking tray with baking paper. Place the quinoa balls onto the lined baking tray and drizzle a little olive oil over the top.

Bake in the oven at 180°C for 10 MIN, then turn each one over and cook for another 10 MIN. Once each side has browned, remove from the oven and set aside.

TUSCAN SAUCE

Traditional ~ Peel and finely dice the onion and garlic. Slice the celery and grate the carrot. Add the onion, garlic, celery and carrot to a large frypan with the olive oil and sauté over a medium–low heat for 3 MIN. Add the remaining ingredients, then reduce the heat to a simmer and cook for 10 MIN, stirring regularly.

Thermomix ~ Roughly chop the celery and carrot. Add these plus the peeled onion and garlic to the cleaned TM bowl. Chop for 4 SEC / SP 6. Scrape down the sides of the bowl, then add the olive oil and sauté for 3 MIN / VAROMA / SP 1. Add the remaining ingredients and cook for 10 MIN / 100°C / SP STIR.

~ ~ ~ ~ ~ ~ ~ ~ ~ ~ ~ ~ ~ ~ ~

SPAGHETTI COOKING INSTRUCTIONS

While the sauce is cooking and the quinoa balls are baking, fill a large pot with filtered water and add a pinch of salt. Bring this to the boil, then add the spaghetti and cook as per packet instructions. Drain the excess liquid from the spaghetti.

~ ~ ~ ~ ~ ~ ~ ~ ~ ~ ~ ~ ~ ~ ~

Layer each serving dish with spaghetti, then top with the tuscan quinoa balls and sauce. Sprinkle some cashew parmesan and fresh basil leaves over the top.

NOTES

This meal takes a little longer than most recipes in this book, however it is totally worth the effort.

DINNER

MINESTRONE SOUP

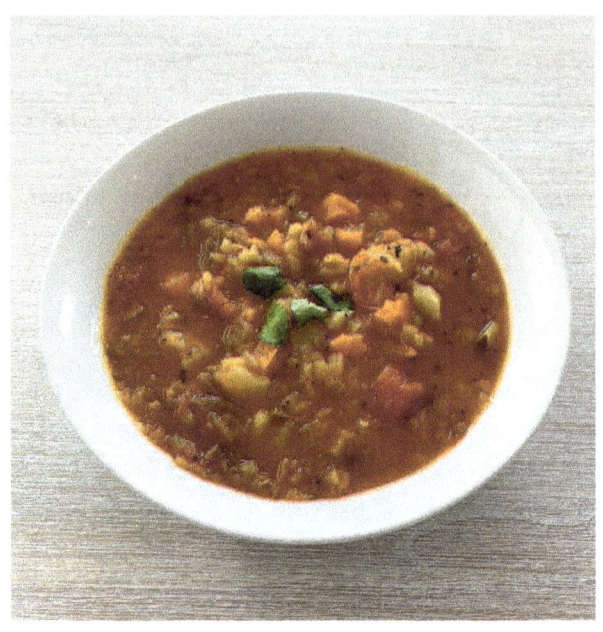

Prep. Time:	Cook Time:	Serves:
15 min	30 min	4

DIRECTIONS

Traditional ~ Peel and finely dice the onion and garlic. Add to a large saucepan along with the dried herbs and olive oil. Sauté over a low heat for 5 MIN.

Wash and dice the vegetables into 1cm cubes and place into the saucepan. Stir to combine then add all the remaining ingredients. Bring this to a boil, then reduce the heat and simmer for 25-30 MIN.

Thermomix ~ Peel the onion and garlic. Cut the onion in half. Add these into the TM bowl and chop for 4 SEC / SP 5. Scrape down the sides of the bowl.

Add the dried herbs and olive oil. Sauté for 3 MIN / VAROMA / SP 1. Roughly cut the zucchini, celery, peeled carrots and potatoes. Add these vegetables into the TM bowl. Chop for 10 SEC / SP 4. Scrape down the sides of the TM bowl.

Add all the remaining ingredients (make sure the water does not go over the max line). Cook for 30 MIN / 100°C / REVERSE / SP 1.

~ ~ ~ ~ ~ ~ ~ ~ ~ ~ ~ ~ ~ ~ ~

Serve in bowls and enjoy.

INGREDIENTS

- 150g (1 medium) Brown Onion
- 3 Garlic Cloves
- 1 tsp dried Basil
- 1 tsp dried Oregano
- 15g (1 Tbsp) Olive Oil
- 140g (½) Zucchini
- 225g (5 sticks) Celery
- 200g (2 medium) Carrots
- 220g (1 medium) Potato
- 40g (2 Tbsp) Vegetable Stock Paste (pg. 65)
- ½ tsp ground Black Pepper
- 15g (1 Tbsp) Organic Tamari Sauce
- 800g (3 ¼ cups) Filtered Water
- 20g (1 Tbsp) Tomato Paste
- 1 x 400g tinned Diced Tomatoes
- 15g (1 Tbsp) French Style Lentils
- 15g (1 Tbsp) Red Split Lentils

NOTES

This soup freezes for up to 1 month in an airtight container.

DINNER

BASIL PESTO PASTA

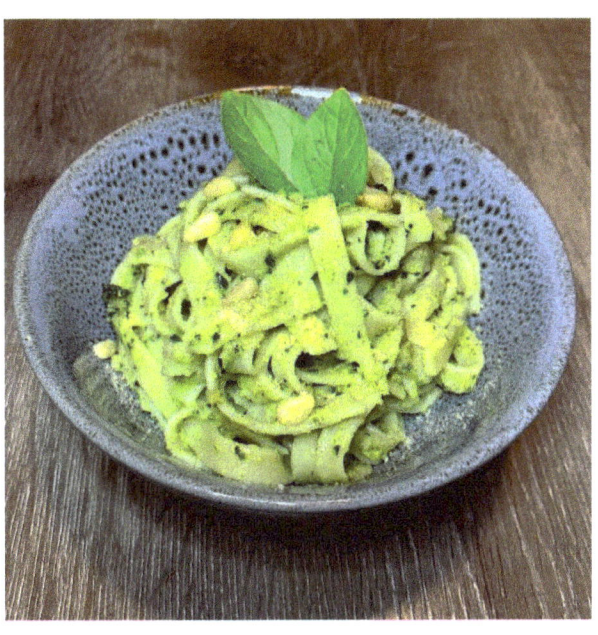

Prep. Time:	Cook Time:	Serves:
5 min	20 min	4

INGREDIENTS

- 250g Fettuccine
- 95g (¾ cup) Unsalted Cashews
- 10g (2 Tbsp) Nutritional Yeast
- 40g (¼ cup) Pine Nuts
- 1 Garlic Clove
- 25g (2 cups loosely packed) Fresh Basil Leaves
- 110g (½ cup) Olive Oil
- ¼ tsp fine Sea Salt

SERVING

- Extra Fresh Basil Leaves
- Cashew Parmesan (pg. 64)
- Pine Nuts

DIRECTIONS

1. Make the cashew parmesan for serving (pg. 64).

2. Fill a large saucepan with filtered water, add a pinch of salt and bring to the boil. Break the dried fettuccine in half and place into the boiling water. Cook as per packet instructions. Once cooked, drain the pasta and return it to the empty pot.

Traditional ~ Add the cashews and nutritional yeast into a food processor or blender and blitz on high. Wash and pat dry the basil leaves. Add the basil leaves plus all remaining ingredients. Chop or pulse on a medium speed until a pesto is formed.

Thermomix ~ Add the cashews and nutritional yeast into the TM bowl and blitz for 5 SEC / SP 9. Wash and pat dry the basil leaves. Add the basil leaves plus the remaining ingredients and chop for 20 SEC / SP 5.

~~~~~~~~~~~~~~~

Add the Basil Pesto to the saucepan of drained pasta and stir over a low heat for 1-2 MIN.

Serve in bowls and sprinkle with the cashew parmesan, fresh basil leaves and pine nuts.

NOTES

The pesto can be used as a dip as well.

If storing for a later date, place the pesto into a clean glass jar and cover the top with a layer of olive oil. Seal and store in the fridge for up to 1 month.

DINNER

NOURISH STEW

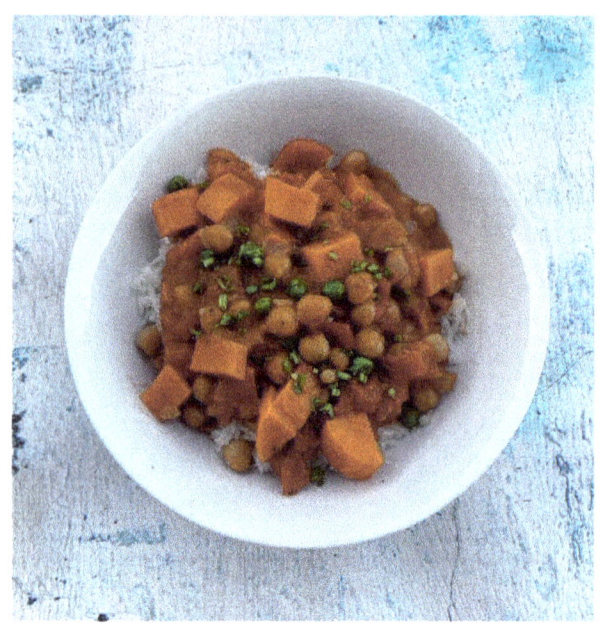

Prep. Time:	Cook Time:	Serves:
10 min	23 min	4

INGREDIENTS

- 200g (1 cup) Organic Basmati Rice
- 75g (½ medium) Brown Onion
- 3 Garlic Cloves
- 2cm cube fresh Ginger
- 15g (1 Tbsp) Olive Oil
- 300g (¾ medium) Sweet Potato
- 230g (2) Roma Tomatoes
- 2 tsp Garam Masala Powder
- ½ tsp ground Cumin
- ¼ tsp ground Black Pepper
- 20g (1 Tbsp) Vegetable Stock Paste (pg. 65)
- Handful of fresh Coriander Leaves
- 1 x 400g tinned Diced Tomatoes
- 1 x 400ml tinned Organic Coconut Cream
- Juice of ½ fresh Lime
- 35g (¼ cup) Frozen Peas
- 1 x 400g tinned Chickpeas

DIRECTIONS

1. Rinse the rice under water using a sieve. Add to a small saucepan with 1 ½ cups filtered water. Cover and bring to the boil, then simmer for 10 MIN or until the water is absorbed. For the TM method see pg. 5 – this just extends the overall time of the recipe.

Traditional ~ Peel and finely dice the onion, garlic and ginger. Add to a large frypan (with a lid) along with the olive oil. Sauté for 2 MIN.

Peel and dice the sweet potato into 2cm cubes. Cut each tomato into 8 pieces. Add the sweet potato, tomatoes, garam masala, cumin powder, black pepper, vegetable stock paste, coriander leaves, tinned tomatoes, tin of coconut cream and lime juice to the frypan. Stir together. Place the lid on and turn the heat to medium-low. Cook for 20 MIN stirring occasionally. Add the frozen peas and drained chickpeas. Stir for 2 MIN.

Thermomix ~ Peel the onion, garlic and ginger. Place these into the TM bowl and chop for 1 SEC / SP 7. Scrape down the sides of the bowl. Add the olive oil and sauté for 3 MIN / VAROMA / SP STIR.

Peel and roughly chop the sweet potato. Add to the TM bowl. Chop for 5 SEC / SP 4. Cut each Roma tomato into 8 pieces. Add to the TM bowl with the garam masala, cumin powder, black pepper, vegetable stock paste, coriander leaves, tinned tomatoes, tin of coconut cream and lime juice.

Cook for 18 MIN / 120°C / REVERSE / SP 1. Add the frozen peas and drained chickpeas and cook for 2 MIN / 120°C / REVERSE / SP STIR.

~ ~ ~ ~ ~ ~ ~ ~ ~ ~ ~ ~ ~ ~

Serve in bowls over the cooked rice.

DINNER

ROAST PUMPKIN RISOTTO

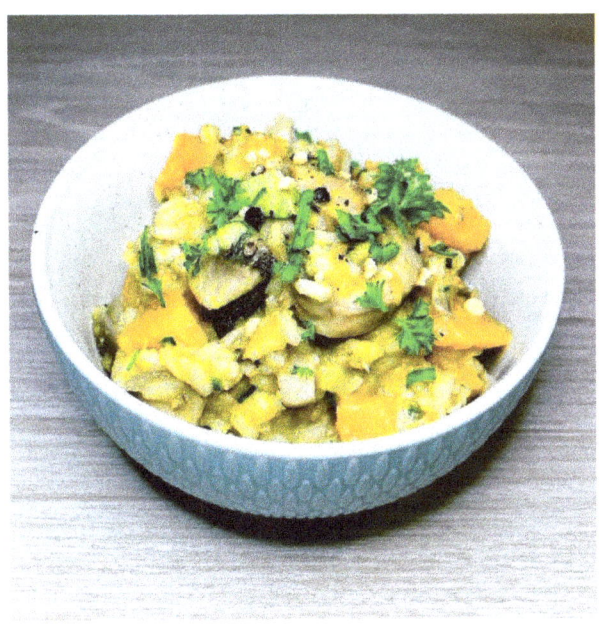

INGREDIENTS

- 600g (½) Butternut Pumpkin
- 75g (½ medium) Red Onion
- 3 Garlic Cloves
- 140g (½) Zucchini
- 110g (2 large) Brown Mushrooms
- 15g (1 Tbsp) Olive Oil
- 260g (1 ¼ cups) Arborio Rice
- 600g (2 ½) cups Filtered Water
- 50g (2 ½ Tbsp) Vegetable Stock Paste (pg. 65)
- 35g (¼ cup) Cashew Parmesan (pg. 64)
- 30g (2 Tbsp) Organic Coconut Cream
- 10g (2 Tbsp) Nutritional Yeast
- Handful of Fresh Parsley
- Handful of Fresh Garlic Chives

SERVING

- Fresh Parsley Leaves
- Fresh Garlic Chives

DINNER

ROAST PUMPKIN RISOTTO (CONTINUED)

Prep. Time: 15 min   Cook Time: 25-35 min   Serves: 4

DIRECTIONS

1. Peel and dice the pumpkin into 1cm cubes. Place onto a lined baking tray. Drizzle a little olive oil over the top. Season with salt and pepper. Bake in the oven for 20 MIN.

Traditional ~ In a small saucepan, add the water and vegetable stock paste and bring to a simmer.

Peel and finely dice the onion and garlic. Place these into a large saucepan. Quarter and finely slice the zucchini, add it to the saucepan along with the olive oil. Over a medium heat, sauté for 5 MIN.

Add the rice and stir for 2 MIN. Add the sliced mushrooms and stir to combine.

Add 1 ladle spoon of stock liquid, into the saucepan with the rice and vegetables. Stir briefly and allow the rice to absorb the liquid. Repeat this process (1 ladle spoon at a time) until all the stock liquid has been absorbed by the rice mixture. This should take around 20–25 MIN.

Add the roast pumpkin from the oven, along with the cashew parmesan, coconut cream, nutritional yeast and finely chopped herbs. Gently stir together for 2 MIN.

Thermomix ~ Peel the onion and garlic. Add these into the TM bowl. Chop for 1 SEC / SP 7. Roughly cut the zucchini and add into the TM bowl. Chop for 4 SEC / SP 4. Scrape down the sides of the TM bowl. Add the olive oil and sauté for 3 MIN / VAROMA / REVERSE / SP STIR.

Add the rice and sauté for 3 MIN / VAROMA / REVERSE / SP 1, placing the simmering basket instead of the measuring cup on top of the mixing bowl lid.

Scrape the bottom of the TM bowl. Add the sliced mushrooms, water and stock paste. Cook for 8 MIN / 100°C / REVERSE / SP 1, placing the simmering basket on top of the lid again.

Add the cashew parmesan, coconut cream, nutritional yeast and finely chopped herbs. Cook for 2 MIN / 100°C / REVERSE / SP 1, placing the simmering basket on top of the lid. Add the roast pumpkin and gently stir through using a spatula.

~ ~ ~ ~ ~ ~ ~ ~ ~ ~ ~ ~ ~ ~ ~

Serve in bowls and garnish with extra parsley and garlic chives.

DINNER

FALAFELS

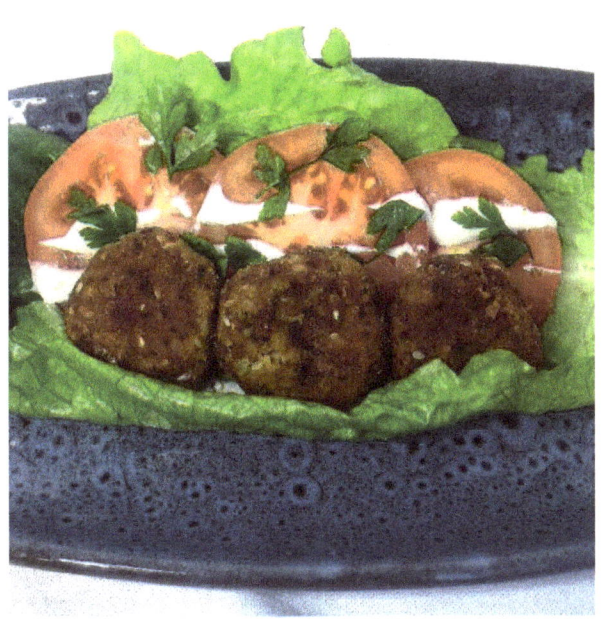

INGREDIENTS

- 1 x 400g tinned Chickpeas
- 75g (½ medium) Brown Onion
- 4 Garlic Cloves
- 5g (¼ cup) fresh Parsley Leaves-loosely packed
- 15g (1 Tbsp) Organic Coconut Oil
- ½ tsp ground Black Pepper
- ½ tsp fine Sea Salt
- 10g (1 Tbsp) Sesame Seeds
- 10g (2 tsp) Sweet Chilli Sauce
- 5g (2 tsp) ground Cumin
- 1 tsp dried Coriander
- ¼ tsp ground Paprika
- 40g (¼ cup) Coconut Flour

SERVING

- Cos Lettuce Leaves
- Tomato slices
- Cashew Aioli (pg. 67)

Prep. Time: 10 min
Cook Time: 30 min
Makes: 12 balls

DIRECTIONS

1. Rinse and thoroughly pat dry the chickpeas. Remove and discard all the chickpea skins. Set aside the chickpeas.

Traditional ~ Peel and roughly cut the onion and garlic. Add to a food processor along with the parsley and dry chickpeas. Blitz together until combined. Add the remaining ingredients and mix until a thick paste like consistency forms.

Thermomix ~ Peel the onion and garlic. Add the onion, garlic, parsley and dry chickpeas to the TM bowl. Blitz together for 3 SEC / SP 10. Scrape down the sides of the bowl. Add the remaining ingredients and mix for 10 SEC / SP 4.

~ ~ ~ ~ ~ ~ ~ ~ ~ ~ ~ ~ ~ ~ ~

Line a baking tray with baking paper. Using a small bowl of water, wet your hands and roll the falafel mix into balls. Place the falafels evenly onto the tray and flatten slightly.

Drizzle some olive oil lightly over the top of each falafel.

Bake in the oven at 180°C for 15 MIN, then carefully flip each one over and bake for another 15 MIN.

While baking, prepare the serving ingredients.

~ ~ ~ ~ ~ ~ ~ ~ ~ ~ ~ ~ ~ ~ ~

Serve the falafels inside each lettuce leaf. Layer with tomato slices and drizzle with cashew aioli.

DINNER

OVEN VEGETABLE BAKE

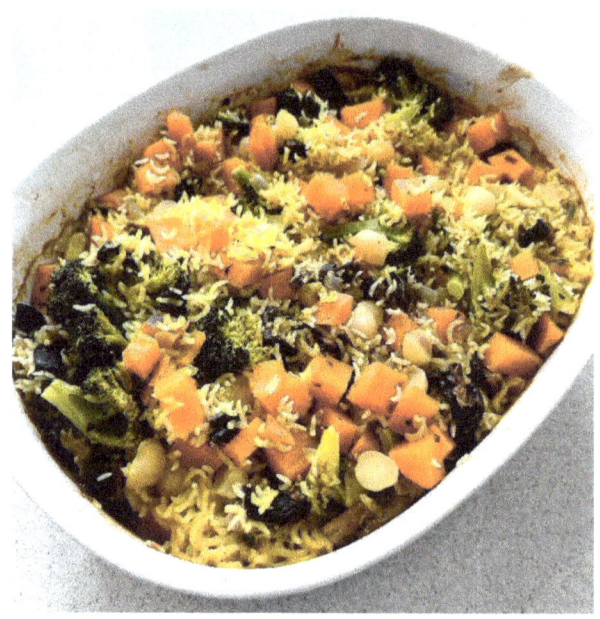

Prep. Time: 10 min **Cook Time:** 1 hr **Serves:** 4

DIRECTIONS – Traditional Only

Traditional ~ Peel and finely dice the onion. Peel and cut the sweet potato into 2cm cubes. Slice the mushrooms and broccoli into small pieces. Add the onion, sweet potato, mushrooms and broccoli to a large casserole dish (with a lid).

Using a sieve, rinse the rice under water until the liquid turns clear then add it into the casserole dish.

Roughly chop the macadamia nuts and add these plus all the remaining ingredients into the casserole dish. Stir gently until combined. Place the casserole lid on.

Bake in the oven at 180°C for 1 HOUR.

~ ~ ~ ~ ~ ~ ~ ~ ~ ~ ~ ~ ~ ~ ~

Serve and enjoy.

INGREDIENTS

- 75g (½ medium) Red Onion
- 400g (1 medium) Sweet Potato
- 80g (2 large) Swiss Brown Mushrooms
- 100g (1 ¾ cup) Broccoli
- 200g (1 cup) Organic Basmati Rice
- 70g (½ cup) Unsalted Macadamia Nuts
- 1 x 400ml tinned Organic Coconut Cream
- 315g (1 ¼ cups) Filtered Water
- 20g (1 Tbsp) Vegetable Stock Paste (pg. 65)
- 5g (1 tsp) Organic Tamari Sauce
- Handful of Coriander Leaves
- 10g (1 Tbsp) Indian Curry Powder (optional)

DINNER

STIR FRY ASIAN NOODLES

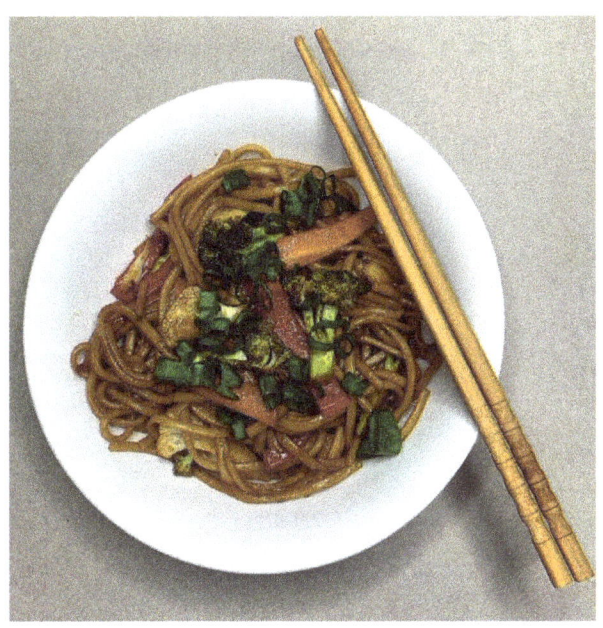

Prep. Time: 10 min   Cook Time: 25 min   Serves: 4

DIRECTIONS – Traditional Only

Traditional ~ Slice the cauliflower and broccoli into florets. Halve and thinly slice the zucchini and capsicum. Cut the eggplant into 1cm cubes. Peel and thinly slice the carrots.

Line a baking tray with baking paper. Spread the vegetables out, then drizzle with olive oil and season with salt and pepper.

Bake in the oven at 180°C for 25 MIN.

In a medium sized bowl, add the sauce ingredients and stir together, then set aside.

In a small saucepan, bring 1L of filtered water to the boil. Snap the udon noodles in half and turn the heat to medium-low. Add the noodles to the water and cook for 10 MIN. Once cooked, drain and set aside.

Once the vegetables have roasted, get a large frypan and add the vegetables, noodles and sauce. Stir for 2-5 MIN over a medium heat.

~ ~ ~ ~ ~ ~ ~ ~ ~ ~ ~ ~ ~ ~ ~

Serve immediately. Garnish with sesame seeds.

INGREDIENTS

- 180g (¼) Cauliflower
- 180g (¼) Broccoli
- 140g (½) Zucchini
- 150g (½ medium) Eggplant
- 75g (½ medium) Red Capsicum
- 200g (2 medium) Carrots
- 15g (1 Tbsp) Olive Oil
- Pinch of fine Sea Salt and ground Black Pepper
- 250g Organic Udon Noodles
- 1L Filtered Water

SAUCE

- 70g (¼ cup) Organic Tamari Sauce
- 60g (⅓ cup) Coconut Sugar
- Juice of ½ fresh Lime
- 10g (2 tsp) Sriracha Chilli Sauce

SERVING

- Sesame Seeds

DINNER

NACHOS

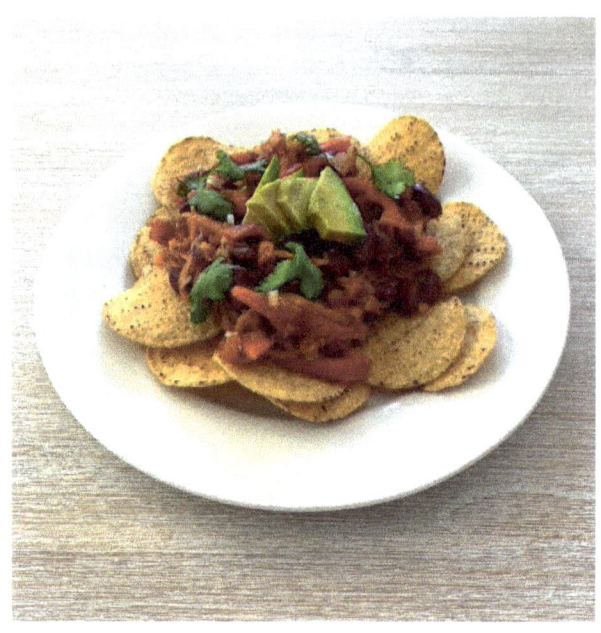

Prep. Time: 10 min
Cook Time: 13 min
Serves: 4

DIRECTIONS

Traditional ~ Peel and finely dice the onion and garlic. Slice the capsicum thinly. Place these into a large frypan, along with the olive oil and sauté over a medium–low heat for 3 MIN.

Grate the carrot and zucchini (squeeze out any excess liquid from the zucchini with some paper towel). Add these to the frypan and stir to combine. Add the tinned tomatoes, tomato paste, mexican spice mix, fresh coriander, and the rinsed and drained beans. Cook for 8 MIN, stirring gently over a medium–low heat.

Thermomix ~ Peel the onion and garlic and place into the TM bowl. Chop for 1 SEC / SP 7. Scrape down the sides of the bowl. Add the olive oil and sauté for 3 MIN / VAROMA / SP 1.

Roughly cut the capsicum, zucchini, carrot and add to the TM bowl. Chop for 10 SEC / SP 4 (*see notes for a hidden vegetable option). Add the tinned tomatoes, tomato paste, mexican spice mix, fresh coriander and the rinsed and drained beans to the TM bowl. Cook for 10 MIN / 100°C / REVERSE / SP 2.

~ ~ ~ ~ ~ ~ ~ ~ ~ ~ ~ ~ ~ ~ ~

Place the corn chips onto each plate, followed by the nacho mix. Top with avocado slices and fresh coriander leaves.

INGREDIENTS

- 15g (1 Tbsp) Organic Coconut Oil
- 75g (½ medium) Brown Onion
- 2 Garlic Cloves
- 125g (½) Red Capsicum
- 140g (½) Zucchini
- 100g (1 medium) Carrot
- 1 x 400g tinned Diced Tomatoes
- 20g (1 Tbsp) Tomato Paste
- 10g (1 Tbsp) Mexican Spice Mix (pg. 69)
- Handful of fresh Coriander Leaves
- 1 x 400g tinned Organic Kidney Beans

SERVING

- Organic Corn Chips
- 1 Avocado (sliced)
- Fresh Coriander leaves
- Cashew Sour Cream (pg. 66) – Optional or make a quick Vegan Sour Cream with ¾ cup Coconut Greek Yoghurt, 2 tsp fresh Lemon Juice and ¼ tsp fine Sea Salt

NOTES

*Hidden vegetable option in the Thermomix (so young kids won't be able to see the vegetables). After adding the roughly chopped capsicum, zucchini and carrot to the TM bowl, chop for 4 SEC / SP 5, then carry on the with the remaining instructions.

DINNER

HEARTY NOODLE SOUP

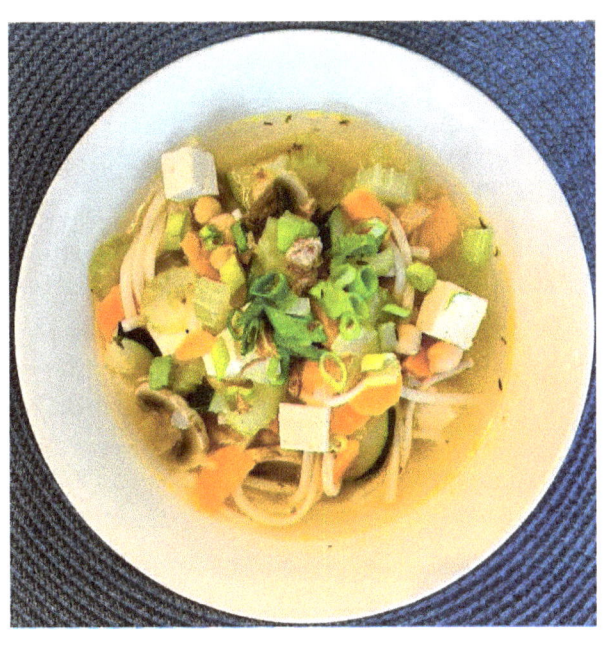

Prep. Time: 10 min **Cook Time:** 30 min **Serves:** 4

INGREDIENTS

- 75g (½ medium) Brown Onion
- 3 Garlic Cloves
- 15g (1 Tbsp) Organic Coconut Oil
- 400g (4 medium) Carrots
- 270g (6 Sticks) of Celery
- ¼ tsp ground Black Pepper
- ½ tsp dried Thyme
- 40g (2 Tbsp) Vegetable Stock Paste (pg. 65)
- 2000g (2L) Filtered Water
- 140g (½) Zucchini
- 80g Organic Tofu
- 1 x 400g tinned Chickpeas
- 60g (2) Button Mushrooms
- 130g Organic Udon Noodles
- Handful of Fresh Bean Sprouts

SERVING

- Handful of fresh Coriander Leaves

DIRECTIONS

Traditional ~ Peel and finely dice the onion and garlic. Peel the carrot, then finely slice the carrot and celery. Add the onion, garlic and coconut oil into a large saucepan. Sauté for 2 MIN over a medium-low heat. Add the carrots, celery, thyme and pepper. Stir together. Cover and cook for 5 MIN (stirring occasionally). Add the water plus vegetable stock paste and bring to a boil. Reduce the heat to low and simmer for 10 MIN.

Rinse and drain the chickpeas. Quarter and thinly slice the zucchini. Slice the mushrooms. Snap the noodles in half. Cut the tofu into 2cm cubes. Add these to the saucepan. Cover and cook over a medium-low heat for 10 MIN, stirring regularly.

Turn off the heat and stir through the bean sprouts.

Thermomix ~ Peel the garlic, onion and carrot. Add the garlic and onion to the TM bowl and chop 1 SEC / SP 7. Scrape down the sides of the bowl. Add the oil and sauté for 2 MIN / VAROMA / SP 1.

Finely slice the carrots and celery. Add to the TM bowl with the thyme and pepper. Cook for 4 MIN / 100°C / REVERSE / SP 1. Add the water and vegetable stock paste. Cook for 10 MIN / 100°C / REVERSE / SP 1.

Rinse and drain the chickpeas. Quarter and thinly slice the zucchini. Slice the mushrooms. Snap the noodles in half and cut the tofu into 2cm cubes. Add these to the TM bowl and cook for 8 MIN / 100°C / REVERSE / SP 1. Add the bean sprouts and cook for 2 MIN / 100°C / REVERSE / SP 1.

~ ~ ~ ~ ~ ~ ~ ~ ~ ~ ~ ~ ~ ~

Serve and sprinkle with fresh coriander.

DINNER

VEGETABLE LAKSA

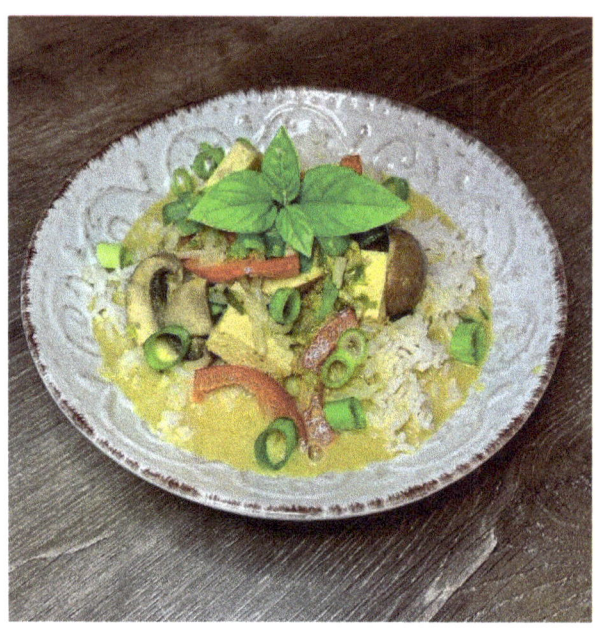

Prep. Time:	Cook Time:	Serves:
10 min	15 min	4

DIRECTIONS

1. Rinse the rice under water using a sieve. Add to a small saucepan along with 1 ½ cups of filtered water. Cover and bring to the boil, then simmer for 10 MIN or until the water is absorbed. For TM method see pg. 5 – this just extends the overall time of the recipe.

Traditional ~ Peel the garlic. Finely dice the garlic, lemongrass and chilli. Add to a large deep saucepan with the coconut oil. Stir over a medium heat until fragrant. Add the curry pastes, coconut cream, lime juice, sugar and tamari sauce. Stir and reduce the heat to a simmer. Add the sliced capsicum, mushrooms and spring onions, cubed tofu and bean sprouts. Cook for 5–10 MIN.

Thermomix ~ Roughly chop the lemongrass. Add to TM bowl with the peeled garlic cloves. Chop for 3 SEC / SP 7. Add the coconut oil and sauté for 3 MIN / VAROMA / SP STIR. Add the curry pastes, coconut cream, lime juice, sugar and tamari sauce. Cook for 8 MIN / 100˚C / SP STIR.

Slice the capsicum and mushrooms. Cut the tofu into 1cm cubes. Add to the TM bowl with the bean sprouts and sliced spring onions. Cook for 5 MIN / 100˚C / REVERSE / SP 1.

~ ~ ~ ~ ~ ~ ~ ~ ~ ~ ~ ~ ~ ~ ~

Serve the laksa over the cooked rice. Garnish with extra sliced spring onions.

NOTES

You can substitute the bean sprouts for a tin of (rinsed and drained) bamboo shoot slices.

INGREDIENTS

- 200g (1 cup) Organic Basmati Rice
- 15g (1 Tbsp) Organic Coconut Oil
- 4 Garlic Cloves
- 1 fresh Lemongrass Stalk
- Fresh Chilli (optional)
- 30g (1 heaped Tbsp) Vegan Red Curry Paste
- 40g (2 Tbsp) Vegan Laksa Curry Paste
- 2 x 400ml tinned Organic Coconut Cream
- Juice of ½ fresh Lime
- 1 tsp Coconut Sugar
- 25g (1 ½ Tbsp) Organic Tamari Sauce
- 125g (½) Red Capsicum
- 60g (2) Button Mushrooms
- 200g Organic Tofu
- 100g Fresh Bean Sprouts
- 2 stalks Spring Onions (green part only) + extra for serving

DINNER

SPICED VEGE SOUP

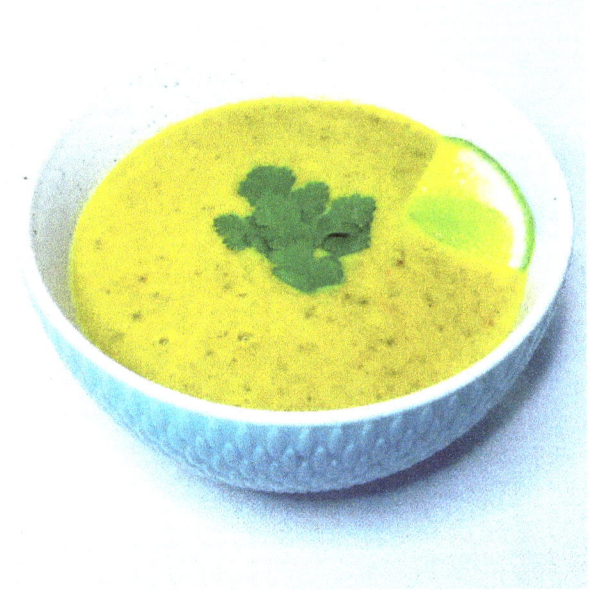

Prep. Time:	Cook Time:	Serves:
10 min	20 min	4

DIRECTIONS

1. Rinse the rice under water using a sieve. Add to a small saucepan along with 1 ½ cups filtered water. Cover and bring to the boil, then simmer for 10 MIN or until the water is absorbed. For TM method see pg. 5 – this just extends the overall time of the recipe.

Traditional ~ Peel the garlic, onion and carrot. Finely dice the garlic, onion, carrot, celery and lemongrass. Add these to a large saucepan (with a lid), along with the coconut oil and pepper. Stir over a medium heat for 2 MIN.

Dice the mushrooms and tomato. Add these plus the remaining ingredients into the saucepan and stir for 3 MIN. Then cover and simmer for 15 MIN. Blend with a stick mixer to get a smooth soup consistency.

Thermomix ~ Peel the onion, garlic and carrot. Roughly cut the carrot, celery and lemongrass. Place the onion, garlic, carrot, celery and lemongrass into the TM bowl. Chop for 4 SEC / SP 5. Add the pepper and coconut oil. Sauté for 3 MIN / VAROMA / SP 1.

Roughly chop the mushrooms and quarter the tomato. Add these plus the remaining ingredients into the TM bowl and cook for 15 MIN / VAROMA / REVERSE / SP 2. Once cooked, blend for 1 MIN / SP 4 gradually working up to SP 9.

~ ~ ~ ~ ~ ~ ~ ~ ~ ~ ~ ~ ~ ~ ~

Serve the soup in bowls over the cooked rice and garnish with the extra coriander leaves.

INGREDIENTS

- 200g (1 cup) Organic Basmati Rice
- 15g (1 Tbsp) Organic Coconut Oil
- 100g (1 medium) Carrot
- 45g (1 stick) Celery
- 75g (½ medium) Brown Onion
- 1 fresh stalk of Lemongrass
- 3 Garlic Cloves
- ½ tsp ground Black Pepper
- 120g (4) Button Mushrooms
- 120g (1) Fresh Tomato
- 5g (½ Tbsp) Curry Powder
- 250g (1 cup) Filtered Water
- 40g (2 Tbsp) Vegetable Stock Paste (pg. 65)
- 20g (1 Tbsp) Pure Maple Syrup
- ¼ tsp Turmeric Powder
- 1 x 400ml tinned Organic Coconut Cream
- Handful of fresh Coriander + extra for serving
- Juice of ¼ fresh Lime

DINNER

CHICKPEA CORN BOWL

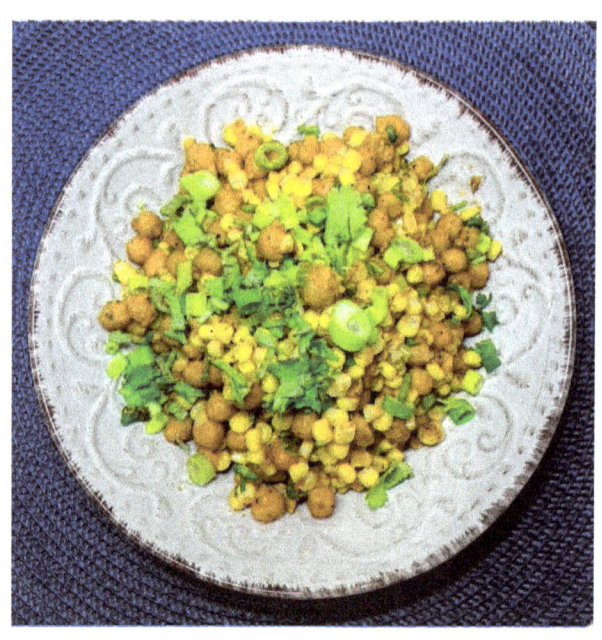

Prep. Time: 10 min
Cook Time: 10 min
Serves: 4

DIRECTIONS – Traditional Only

1. Rinse, drain and pat dry the chickpeas. Remove and discard all the chickpea skins. Set aside the chickpeas.
2. Remove any husks from the corn and slice off the kernels.

Traditional ~ Add the corn to a large frypan with the olive oil and cook on high for 5 MIN or until golden brown.

Turn the heat to low. Slice the spring onions and add to the frypan along with all the remaining ingredients, including the rinsed and drained chickpeas. Stir for 2-5 MIN.

~~~~~~~~~~~~~~

Serve and sprinkle the extra spring onion slices over the top.

INGREDIENTS

- 2 x 400g tinned Organic Chickpeas
- 4 fresh Corn on the Cob
- 30g (2 Tbsp) Olive Oil
- 15g (3 Tbsp) Nutritional Yeast
- 20g (2 Tbsp) Mexican Spice Mix (pg. 69)
- 2 tsp Coconut Sugar
- 1 tsp ground Cumin
- 1 tsp Onion Powder
- Juice of 1 fresh Lime
- 2 stalks Spring Onions (green part only)
- 2 Tbsp fresh Coriander Leaves

SERVING

- Spring Onion (green part only)

DINNER

MAPLE ROASTED COUSCOUS SALAD

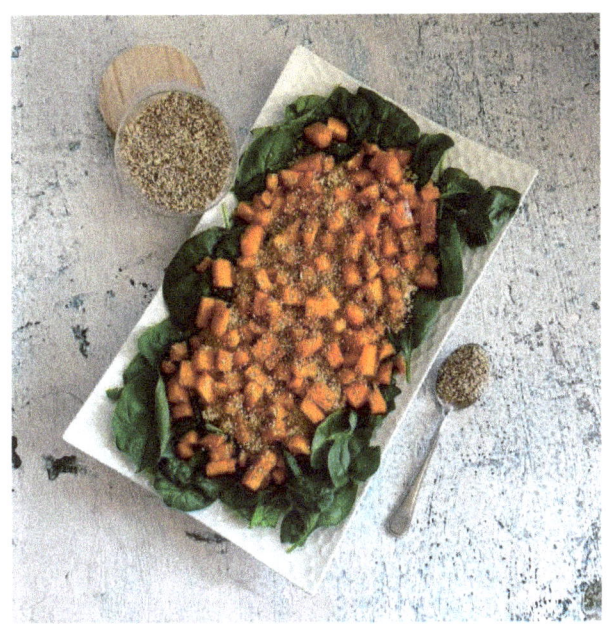

Prep. Time:	Cook Time:	Serves:
15 min	55 min	6+

DIRECTIONS – Traditional Only

Traditional ~ Peel and cut the vegetables into 2cm cubes and place onto a baking tray lined with baking paper. Drizzle the olive oil and maple syrup over the top. Sprinkle the pepper over the vegetables. Gently toss to coat and spread evenly on the tray. Bake in the oven at 200°C for 35–40 MIN.

Place the water, olive oil, salt and pepper into a small saucepan and bring to the boil, then turn the heat off. Add the couscous to the saucepan and place the lid on. Allow this to sit for 5 MIN, then fluff it up with a fork and set aside.

Line another baking tray with baking paper and place all the dukkha ingredients on. Toss and spread evenly on the tray. Place into the oven alongside the vegetables and bake for 5 MIN.

Allow the dukkha to cool, then place it in a food processor and chop until it is a fine crumb consistency. Alternatively chop finely, using a knife or the Thermomix.

Thermomix ~ (Dukkha Only)
Add the roasted dukkha ingredients into the TM and chop for 10 SEC / SP 6.

~ ~ ~ ~ ~ ~ ~ ~ ~ ~ ~ ~ ~ ~ ~

To serve, place the spinach leaves on a large dish, then evenly spread the couscous on, followed by the roasted vegetables. Sprinkle the dukkha over the top.

INGREDIENTS

MAPLE ROASTED VEGETABLES
- 600g (½) large Butternut Pumpkin
- 250g (½ medium) Sweet Potato
- 100g (1 medium) Carrot
- 30g (2 Tbsp) Olive Oil
- 60g (3 Tbsp) Pure Maple Syrup
- ¼ tsp ground Black Pepper
- ¼ tsp fine Sea Salt

COUSCOUS
- 160g (1 cup) Couscous
- 250g (1 cup) Filtered Water
- 15g (1 Tbsp) Olive Oil
- Pinch of fine Sea Salt
- Pinch of ground Black Pepper

DUKKHA
- 10g (1 Tbsp) Natural Almonds
- 35g (¼ cup) Pecans
- 10g (1 Tbsp) Sesame Seeds
- ½ tsp dried Coriander
- ½ tsp ground Cumin
- Pinch of fine Sea Salt

SERVING
- Spinach leaves

NOTES

This makes 55g of dukkha, so you will have some left over to keep for future meals.

DINNER

VEGE ENCHILADAS

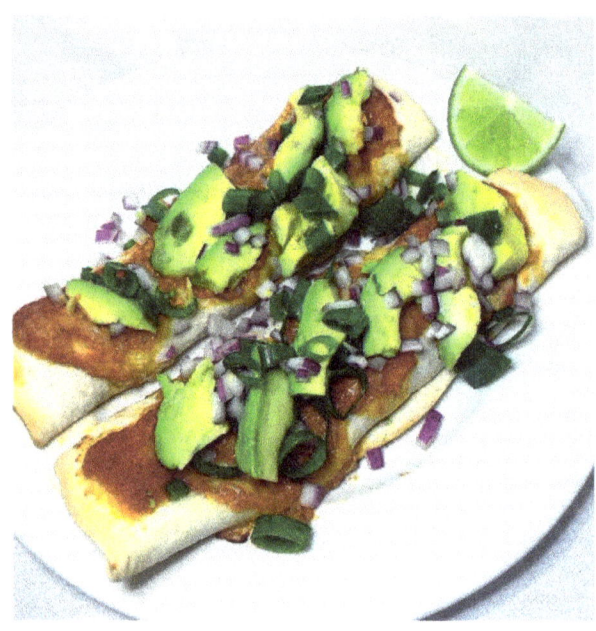

INGREDIENTS

ENCHILADA SAUCE

- 75g (½ medium) Brown Onion
- 4 Garlic Cloves
- 15g (1 Tbsp) Organic Coconut Oil
- 1 x 400g tinned Diced Tomatoes
- 20g (1 Tbsp) Pure Maple Syrup
- 5g (1 tsp) Vegetable Stock Paste (pg. 65)
- 60g (¼ cup) Filtered Water
- 20g (1 Tbsp) Tomato Paste
- 1 tsp ground Paprika
- 1 tsp ground Cumin
- ¼ tsp dried Oregano
- ¼ tsp Garlic Powder
- ¼ tsp fine Sea Salt
- ¼ tsp ground Black Pepper

ENCHILADA FILLING

- 75g (½ medium) Brown Onion
- 120g (1 small) Capsicum
- 60g (2) button Mushrooms
- 140g (½) Zucchini
- 15g (1 Tbsp) Organic Coconut Oil
- 1 x 400g tinned Organic Black Beans
- 125g tinned Corn Kernels

SERVING

- Tortillas
- Avocado
- 2 stalks Spring Onion (green part only)
- ¼ Red Onion
- ½ fresh Lime (cut into wedges)
- Fresh Coriander Leaves

DINNER

VEGE ENCHILADAS (CONTINUED)

Prep. Time: 20 min Cook Time: 40 min Serves: 4

DIRECTIONS

ENCHILADA SAUCE

Traditional ~ Peel and finely dice the onion and garlic. Add these to a frypan with the coconut oil and sauté for 3 MIN.

Add the remaining ingredients to the frypan and cook over a medium heat for 5 MIN, stirring frequently.

Allow to cool slightly and transfer to a heat proof bowl. Using a stick mixer, blend until it becomes a sauce consistency.

Place ⅓ of the sauce into a sperate bowl and set aside. This will be used to spread over the top of the enchiladas before baking.

Thermomix ~ Peel and add the onion and garlic to the TM bowl and chop for 1 SEC / SP 7. Scrape down the sides of the TM bowl and add the coconut oil. Sauté for 3 MIN / VAROMA / SP 1.

Add the remaining ingredients and cook for 5 MIN / 100°C / SP 1. Then blend for 7 SEC / SP 7.

Empty into 2 heat proof bowls, with ⅓ of the sauce in one bowl and ⅔ of the sauce in the other bowl. Set aside. The ⅓ sauce will be used to spread over the top of the enchiladas before baking.

ENCHILADA FILLING

Traditional ~ Rinse and drain the beans and corn. Dice the onion, capsicum, mushrooms and zucchini. Add these plus the coconut oil to a large frypan and cook for 10 MIN or until tender.

Thermomix ~ Rinse and drain the beans and corn. Place the onion, quartered capsicum, mushrooms and roughly chopped zucchini into the TM bowl and chop for 4 SEC / SP 4. Add the beans, corn and coconut oil to the TM bowl and cook for 8 MIN / 90°C / REVERSE / SP STIR.

~~~~~~~~~~~~~~~

ASSEMBLING THE ENCHILADAS

Warm each tortilla in a frypan to soften (this makes them easier to roll). Line a baking tray with baking paper.

Spread the ⅔ bowl of the sauce evenly over each tortilla. Place some of the filling lengthways across each. Then carefully roll, and place (fold side down) on the tray. With the remaining ⅓ sauce, spread a small amount across the top of each tortilla.

Repeat this process until all the tortillas are ready to be baked.

Bake in the oven at 180°C for 20-25 MIN or until slightly browned.

Finely slice the avocado and spring onions. Finely dice the red onion, ready for serving.

Once baked, serve on plates and top with the avocado, spring onions, red onion, coriander leaves and a squeeze of lime juice.

DINNER

SWEET N SOUR CRISPY TOFU

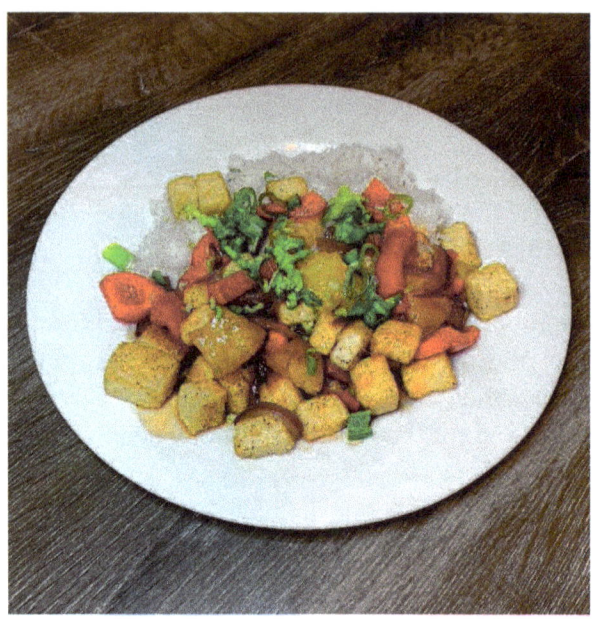

Prep. Time:	Cook Time:	Serves:
15 min	40 min	4

DIRECTIONS – Traditional Only

Traditional ~ Rinse the rice under water using a sieve. Add to a small saucepan with 1 ½ cups filtered water. Cover and bring to the boil, then simmer for 10 MIN or until the water is absorbed.

Slice the tofu into 2cm cubes, then gently press with paper towel to remove any excess liquid.

In a medium sized bowl, add the arrowroot flour, garlic powder and salt. Stir to combine. Then gently toss the tofu to coat in the flour mixture. Add the olive oil to a large frypan. Warm the oil over a medium-high heat, then add the tofu and cook until crispy. Once cooked, place the crispy tofu onto a separate plate and set aside. Clean and dry the frypan.

Pour the liquid from the tinned pineapple into a small saucepan (keeping the pineapple pieces separate). Add the rice wine vinegar, tomato sauce and brown sugar into the saucepan. Turn the heat up high stirring the sauce frequently for 10–15 MIN until you have a thick syrup like sauce. Take off the heat and set aside.

Peel the garlic and ginger. Finely slice the garlic, ginger, red onion and capsicum. Place into the cleaned frypan with the sesame oil. Sauté for 10 MIN over a medium heat. Slice the pineapple and add to the frypan, stirring for another 2 MIN. Then add the crispy tofu and sauce mixture. Reduce the heat to low and stir for 2 MIN.

~ ~ ~ ~ ~ ~ ~ ~ ~ ~ ~ ~ ~ ~ ~

Serve in bowls by adding the cooked rice, followed by the crispy tofu mix. Garnish with fresh coriander leaves.

INGREDIENTS

- 210g (1 cup) Organic Basmati Rice
- 500g Organic Tofu
- 35g (¼ cup) Arrowroot Flour
- 1 tsp Garlic Powder
- ½ tsp fine Sea Salt
- 30g (2 Tbsp) Olive Oil
- 30g (2 Tbsp) Sesame Oil
- 8cm x 2cm piece of fresh Ginger
- 1 Garlic Clove
- 75g (½ medium) Red Onion
- 250g (1 medium) Capsicum
- 1 x 440g tinned Pineapple slices – in juice
- 45g (3 Tbsp) Rice Wine Vinegar
- 60g (3 Tbsp) Tomato Sauce (good quality)
- 40g (¼ cup) Brown Sugar

SERVING

- Handful of fresh Coriander leaves

DINNER

CORIANDER LIME CAULI RICE

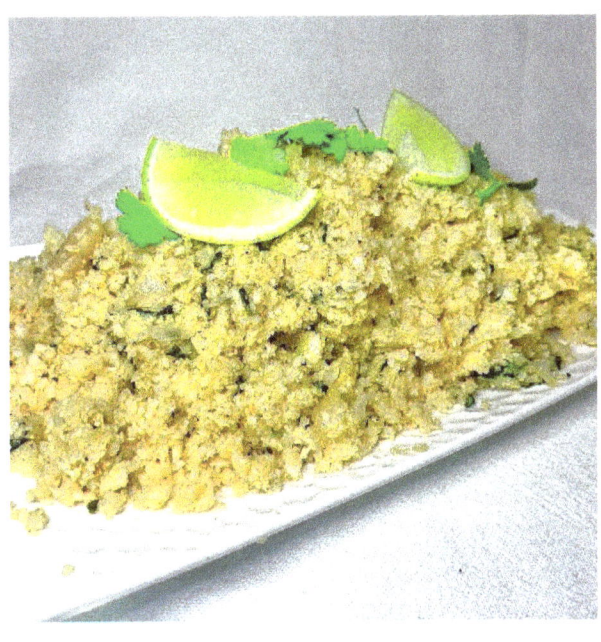

Prep. Time: 10 min **Cook Time:** 15 min **Serves:** 2-4

INGREDIENTS

- 550g (1 whole) Cauliflower, cut into florets
- 15g (1 Tbsp) Organic Coconut Oil
- 2 Garlic Cloves
- 75g (½ medium) Brown Onion
- Juice of 2 fresh Limes
- ¼ cup fresh Coriander
- ¼ tsp ground Black Pepper
- ½ tsp fine Sea Salt
- ½ tsp ground Paprika
- ½ tsp ground Cumin

SERVING

- 1 fresh Lime – cut into wedges
- Fresh Coriander Leaves

DIRECTIONS

Traditional ~ Cut the cauliflower into florets. Place the cauliflower pieces into a food processor and blitz until you have a rice like consistency.

Peel and finely dice the onion and garlic. In a large frypan, melt the coconut oil over a medium heat, then add the onion and garlic and cook for 5 MIN, stirring frequently.

Add the cauliflower rice, lime juice, coriander, pepper, salt, paprika and cumin to the frypan. Stir together. Cover and cook for 5-10 MIN, stirring frequently.

Thermomix ~ Cut the cauliflower into florets. Place the cauliflower pieces into the TM bowl and chop for 3 SEC / SP 9. Empty into a separate large bowl and set aside.

Peel the onion and garlic and add into the TM bowl. Chop for 1 SEC / SP 7. Scrape down the sides of the TM bowl and add the coconut oil. Sauté for 3 MIN / VAROMA / SP 1.

Return the cauliflower back into the TM bowl. Add the lime juice, coriander, pepper, salt, paprika and cumin. Cook for 8 MIN / 90°C / REVERSE / SP STIR.

~~~~~~~~~~~~~~~

Serve immediately. Sprinkle some coriander leaves over the top and add the lime wedges.

NOTES

As a main meal this will feed 2 people and served as a side dish, it will feed 4+ people.

DINNER

BURGER PATTIES

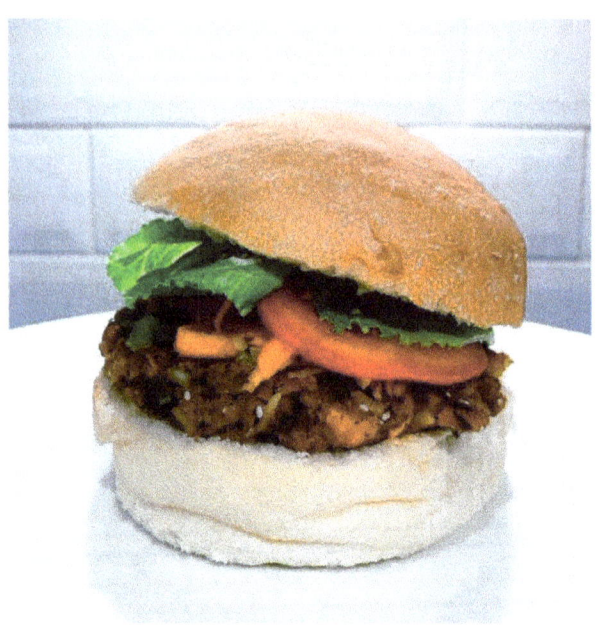

Prep. Time:	Cook Time:	Serves:
15 min	30 min	6

DIRECTIONS

1. Peel and thinly slice the sweet potato. Place onto 2 baking trays lined with baking paper. Drizzle the olive oil over the top and season with the dried rosemary. Gently toss and bake in the oven at 180°C for 15 MIN.

2. Rinse, drain and pat dry the black beans.

Traditional ~ Rinse the rice under water using a sieve. Add to a small saucepan with 1 ½ cups filtered water. Cover and bring to a boil, then reduce the heat to a simmer. Cook for 10 MIN or until all the water is absorbed.

Add the cooked rice and sweet potato into a food processor. Add the black beans and remaining ingredients and mix on a medium–high speed (or mash all together in a large bowl).

Thermomix ~ Add the rice to the simmering basket and rinse under water. Insert the simmering basket into the TM bowl. Add 1000g filtered water. Cook for 15 MIN / 100°C / SP4. Once cooked, remove the simmering basket, discard the liquid. Return the rice to the TM bowl.

Add the cooked sweet potato, black beans and remaining ingredients. Mix for 15 SEC / SP 5. Scrape down the sides of the bowl as needed.

~ ~ ~ ~ ~ ~ ~ ~ ~ ~ ~ ~ ~ ~ ~

Scoop and roll the burger patty mixture into palm sized balls then flatten each slightly. Using a large frypan, add a little olive oil and lightly fry each side.

Add a patty to each bread bun, along with lettuce leaves, sliced avocado and tomato. Add some plant-based aioli and good quality tomato sauce.

INGREDIENTS

- 100g (½ cup) Organic Basmati Rice
- 500g (1 medium) Sweet Potato
- 15g (1 Tbsp) Olive Oil
- 5g (1 Tbsp) dried Rosemary
- 1x 400g tinned Organic Black Beans
- 40g (½ cup) Breadcrumbs
- ½ tsp fine Sea Salt
- ½ tsp ground Black Pepper
- 5g (2 tsp) Garlic Powder
- 5g (2 tsp) ground Paprika
- 5g (2 tsp) ground Cumin
- 10g (2 tsp) Chia Seeds

SERVING

- Bread Buns
- Lettuce
- Avocado
- Tomato

DINNER

EGGPLANT PARMIGANA

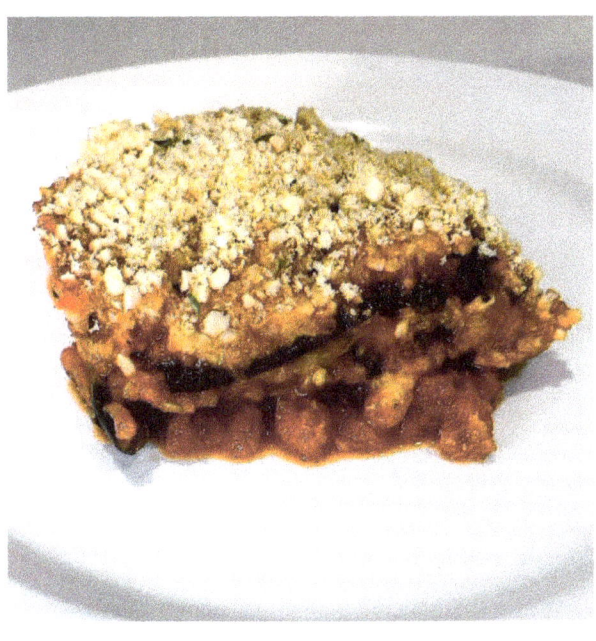

Prep. Time:	Cook Time:	Serves:
10 min	45 min	4

DIRECTIONS

1. Wash and cut the eggplant into 1cm thick slices. Line 2 baking trays with baking paper. Place the eggplant slices on evenly. Season with salt and pepper. Bake in the oven at 200°C for 30 MIN. After 15 MIN, turn each piece over.

Traditional ~ Peel and finely dice the onion and garlic. Add to a large saucepan with the olive oil and sauté for 3 MIN. Peel and grate the carrot. Grate the zucchini, removing any excess liquid with paper towel. Add the carrot and zucchini to the saucepan along with the basil, oregano, paprika, tomato paste, vegetable stock paste and passata. Cook for 10 MIN on a medium-low heat.

Thermomix ~ Peel the onion and garlic. Place into the TM bowl and chop for 1 SEC / SP 7. Scrape down the sides of the bowl. Add the olive oil. Sauté for 3 MIN / VAROMA / SP STIR.

Peel the carrot. Roughly cut the carrot and zucchini and add into the TM bowl. Chop for 5 SEC / SP 5. Add the basil, oregano, paprika, tomato paste, vegetable stock paste and passata. Cook for 10 MIN / 100°C / REVERSE / SP 1.

~ ~ ~ ~ ~ ~ ~ ~ ~ ~ ~ ~ ~ ~ ~

Once the eggplant has cooked, remove from the oven and reduce the oven temperature to 180°C. In a small bowl, mix the breadcrumbs and cashew parmesan together.

Using a large lasagne dish begin layering, starting with the sauce, then eggplant, sauce, eggplant. Repeat until the lasagne dish is full. Sprinkle the top layer with the breadcrumb mixture followed by the dried parsley. Bake in the oven at 180°C for 15 MIN.

Allow to cool slightly, then serve.

INGREDIENTS

- 650g (1 large) Eggplant
- 75g (½ medium) Brown Onion
- 2 Garlic Cloves
- 15g (1 Tbsp) Olive Oil
- 160g (2 Medium) Carrots
- 160g (½) Zucchini
- ½ tsp dried Basil
- ½ tsp dried Oregano
- ½ tsp ground Paprika
- 20g (1 Tbsp) Tomato Paste
- 20g (1 Tbsp) Vegetable Stock Paste (pg. 65)
- 1 x 700g jar Passata
- 50g (½ cup) Breadcrumbs
- 70g (½ cup) Cashew Parmesan (pg. 64)
- ½ tsp dried Parsley

DINNER

GREEN CURRY

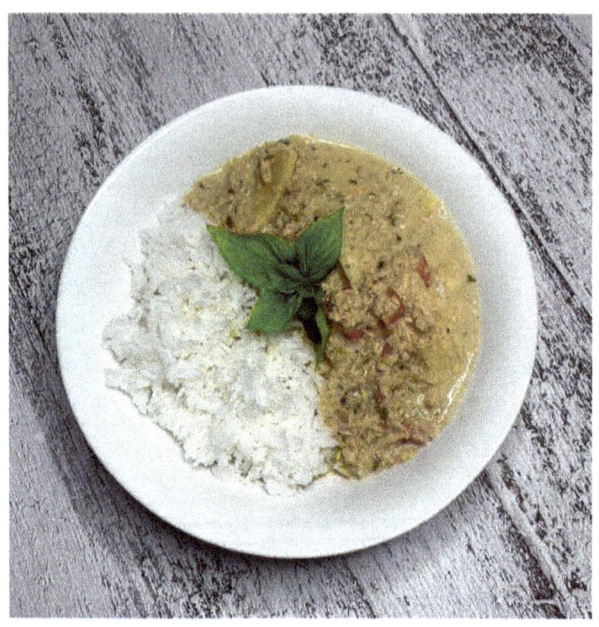

Prep. Time: 10 min   Cook Time: 12 min   Serves: 4

DIRECTIONS

1. Rinse the rice under water, using a sieve. Add to a small saucepan with 1 ½ cups filtered water. Cover and bring to the boil, then simmer for 10 MIN or until the water is absorbed.

Traditional ~ Peel and finely dice the lemongrass, onion, garlic and ginger. Add to a large frypan along with the cumin, sugar, vegetable stock paste, lime juice, tamari sauce, tamarind paste, coriander, basil and cayenne. Stir together and sauté over a low heat for 2 MIN.

Rinse and drain the jackfruit and bamboo slices. Thinly slice the jackfruit and capsicum. Add these plus the coconut cream and water to the frypan and cook for 10 MIN over a medium–low heat, stirring occasionally.

Thermomix ~ Roughly chop the lemongrass then add into the TM bowl along with the peeled onion, garlic and ginger. Add the cumin, sugar, vegetable stock paste, lime juice, tamari sauce, tamarind paste, coriander, basil and cayenne. Mix for 6 SEC / SP 6. Scrape down the sides of the bowl and mix again for 6 SEC / SP 6.

Rinse and drain the jackfruit and bamboo slices. Thinly slice the capsicum. Add the jackfruit to the TM bowl and chop for 4 SEC / SP 4. Rinse and drain the bamboo slice. Add the bamboo slices, capsicum, coconut cream and water to the TM bowl and cook for 8 MIN / 100°C / REVERSE / SP STIR.

~ ~ ~ ~ ~ ~ ~ ~ ~ ~ ~ ~ ~ ~ ~

Serve in bowls over the rice and garnish with fresh basil leaves.

INGREDIENTS

- 200g (1 cup) Organic Basmati Rice
- 1 fresh stalk of Lemongrass
- 75g (½ medium) Red Onion
- 3 Garlic Cloves
- 2 tsp Ginger Powder
- ½ tsp ground Cumin
- 1 tsp Coconut Sugar OR Brown Sugar
- 5g (1 tsp) Vegetable Stock Paste
- Juice of ½ fresh Lime
- 15g (1 Tbsp) Organic Tamari Sauce
- 20g (1 Tbsp) Tamarind Paste
- 5g (1 Tbsp) fresh Coriander
- 5g (2 Tbsp) fresh Basil leaves
- ¼ tsp Cayenne Pepper
- 1 x 400ml tinned Organic Coconut Cream
- 125g (½ cup) Filtered Water
- 1 x 400g tinned Organic Jackfruit
- 125g (½ medium) Red Capsicum
- 1 x 225g tinned Bamboo Shoot Slices

SERVING

- Fresh Basil Leaves

DINNER

CAULIFLOWER BITES

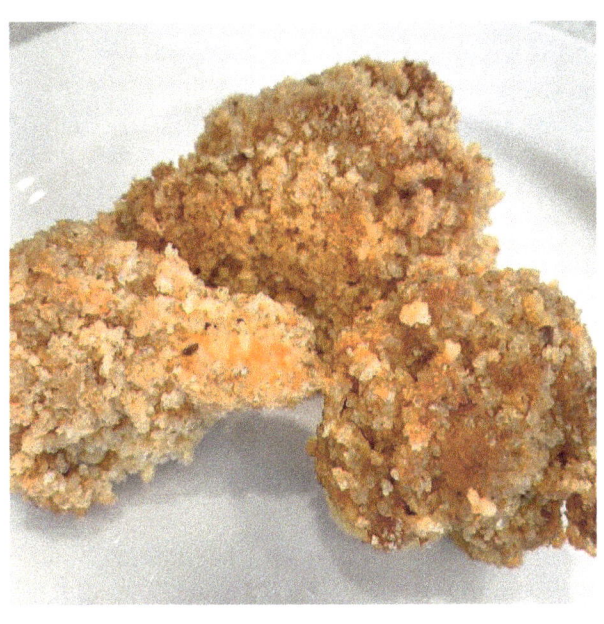

Prep. Time:	Cook Time:	Serves:
10 min	25 min	4

DIRECTIONS

Traditional ~ In a large bowl whisk together the flour, spices, salt, pepper and almond milk to create a batter. In a separate bowl, add the breadcrumbs.

Thermomix ~ Add the flour, spices, salt, pepper and almond milk into the TM bowl. Insert the butterfly attachment. Wisk for 1 MIN / SP 3.

Pour this batter mixture into a large bowl. In a separate bowl, add the breadcrumbs.

~ ~ ~ ~ ~ ~ ~ ~ ~ ~ ~ ~ ~ ~ ~

Cut the entire cauliflower into bite size pieces (including the stems). Dip each piece of cauliflower into the batter mixture, followed by the breadcrumbs. Repeat until all the cauliflower pieces have been coated.

Line 2 baking trays with baking paper. Spread the pieces evenly onto the trays.

Bake at 180°C for 25 MIN.

Serve on plates with cashew aioli sauce.

INGREDIENTS

- 1 whole Cauliflower
- 160g (1 cup) Wholemeal Plain Flour
- 10g (2 tsp) Garlic Powder
- 10g (2 tsp) Onion Powder
- 5g (1 tsp) ground Cumin
- 5g (1 tsp) ground Paprika
- ½ tsp fine Sea Salt
- ½ tsp ground Black Pepper
- ½ tsp dried Parsley
- Pinch of Cayenne Pepper
- 310g (1 ¼ cups) Almond Milk
- 135g (1 ½ cups) Breadcrumbs

SERVING

- Cashew Aioli (pg. 67)

DINNER

SEASONED WEDGES

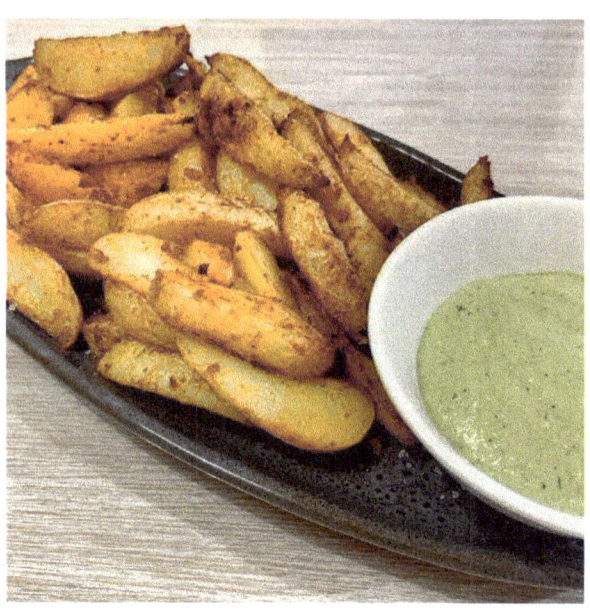

Prep. Time:	Cook Time:	Serves:
10 min	40 min	4

DIRECTIONS

Traditional ~ Wash and cut the potatoes into wedges. Place the potato wedges into a large mixing bowl. Add the olive oil and toss to coat.

In a small separate bowl, add the remaining ingredients. Sprinkle this seasoning mix over the potatoes and gently toss to coat.

Thermomix ~ Wash and cut the potatoes into wedges and place into the TM bowl. Add all the remaining ingredients and mix for 20 SEC / REVERSE / SP 1.

~ ~ ~ ~ ~ ~ ~ ~ ~ ~ ~ ~ ~ ~

Line a baking tray with baking paper and evenly arrange the seasoned potatoes.

Bake in the oven at 180°C for 40 MIN, turning all the wedges over after 20 MIN.

Serve on plates and enjoy with some creamy dill dressing.

INGREDIENTS

- 1kg (approx. 3 large) Potatoes
- 40g (2 ½ Tbsp) Olive Oil
- 10g (2 tsp) ground Paprika
- 10g (2 tsp) Garlic Powder
- 5g (1 tsp) Onion Powder
- ½ tsp dried Oregano
- ¼ tsp ground Cumin
- ½ tsp fine Sea Salt
- Pinch of Cayenne Pepper (optional)

SERVING
- Creamy Dill Dressing (pg. 68)

DINNER

SWEET POTATO PIE

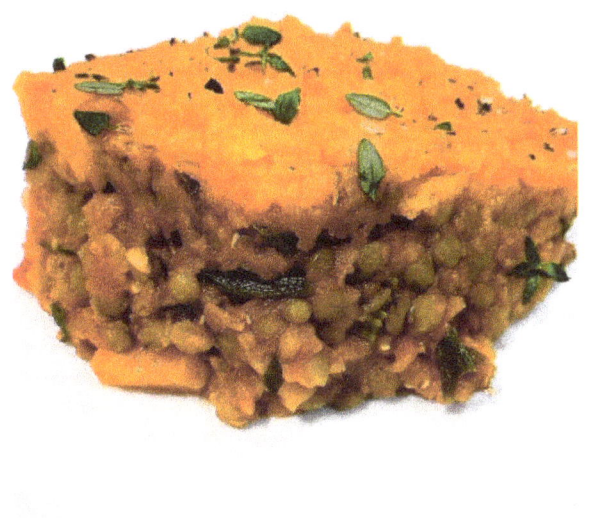

INGREDIENTS

- 750g (1 ½ large) Sweet Potatoes
- 1L (4 cups) Filtered Water
- 1 x 400g tinned Organic Black Lentils
- 15g (1 Tbsp) Olive Oil
- 75g (½ medium) Brown Onion
- 2 Garlic Cloves
- 150 g (2 sticks) Celery
- 200g (2 medium) Carrots
- 60g (1) Portobello Mushroom
- 60g (½ cup) frozen Peas
- 1 x 400g tinned Organic Diced Tomatoes
- 35g (2 Tbsp) Organic Tamari Sauce
- 1 Tbsp fresh Basil Leaves OR 1 tsp dried Basil
- 1 tsp fresh Thyme Leaves OR 1 tsp dried Thyme
- 1 tsp fresh Rosemary Leaves OR 1 tsp dried Rosemary
- 25g (1 cup firmly packed) Spinach Leaves
- 125g (½ cup) Almond Milk
- Pinch of fine Sea Salt
- Pinch of ground Black Pepper

SERVING

- Fresh Thyme leaves

DINNER

SWEET POTATO PIE (CONTINUED)

Prep. Time: 15 min Cook Time: 60 min Serves: 4-6

DIRECTIONS

Traditional ~ In a large saucepan, add the water and bring to the boil. Peel and cut the sweet potatoes into 2cm cubes. Place the sweet potatoes into the boiling water and cook until soft (approx. 20 MIN).

Peel and dice the onion, garlic and carrots. Dice the mushroom. Finely slice the celery. In a large frypan, add these plus the olive oil and stir over a medium heat for 10 MIN.

Rinse and drain the lentils. Add the lentils, frozen peas, tomatoes, tamari sauce, rosemary, thyme and chopped fresh basil to the frypan. Simmer for 10 MIN. Turn off the heat and stir through the roughly chopped spinach leaves.

Drain the liquid from the cooked potatoes. Return the drained potatoes to the saucepan and add the almond milk, salt and pepper. Mash together until smooth.

Thermomix ~ Cut the sweet potato into 2cm cubes and place into the simmering basket. Add 500g water into the TM bowl. Insert the simmering basket and cook for 17 MIN / VAROMA / SP 2.

Remove the simmering basket and set aside to drain. Empty the cooking liquid from the TM bowl. Add the cooked sweet potato back into the TM bowl along with the almond milk, salt and pepper. Blend for 20 SEC / SP 5. Place the mash into the Thermoserver and set aside. Wash and dry the TM bowl.

Peel the onion, garlic and carrots. Roughly cut the celery, carrots and mushroom. Add these plus the onion and garlic to the TM bowl. Chop for 10 SEC / SP 5. Add the oil and cook for 10 MIN / VAROMA / REVERSE / SP 1.

Rinse and drain the lentils. Add the lentils, frozen peas, tomatoes, tamari sauce, rosemary, thyme and chopped fresh basil into the TM bowl. Cook for 5 MIN / 100°C / REVERSE / SP 1.

Add the roughly chopped spinach leaves to the TM bowl. Mix for 20 SEC / REVERSE / SP 3.

~ ~ ~ ~ ~ ~ ~ ~ ~ ~ ~ ~ ~ ~ ~

Pour the cooked pie mixture into a large baking dish. Spread the mash on top. Sprinkle with some fresh thyme leaves and a pinch of salt and pepper.

Bake in the oven at 180°C for 20 MIN.

Allow to cool slightly before slicing and serving on plates.

DINNER

MEXICAN BURRITO BOWL

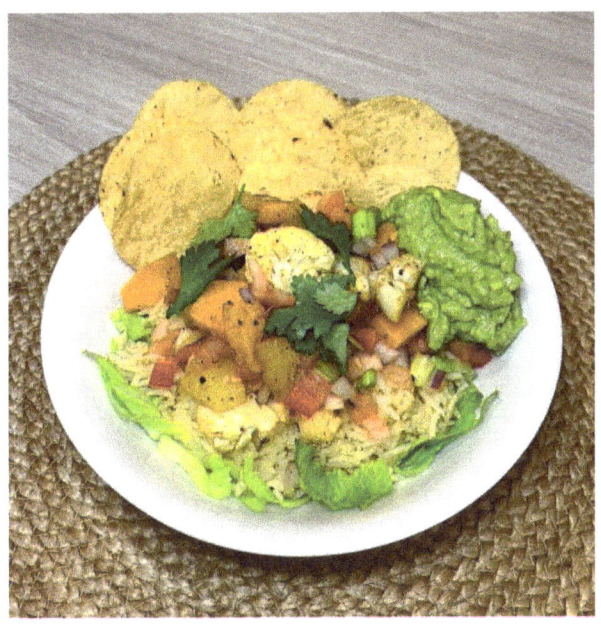

INGREDIENTS

RICE
- 200g (1 cup) Organic Basmati Rice
- 375g (1 ½ cups) Filtered Water
- 20g (1 Tbsp) Vegetable Stock Paste (pg. 65)
- 5g (1 tsp) Mexican Spice Mix (pg. 69)
- Juice of ½ fresh Lime

VEGEATBLE + SALAD MIX
- 500g (1 medium) Sweet Potato
- 180g (¼) Cauliflower
- 1 x 250g tinned Pineapple Slices
- 15g (1 Tbsp) Olive Oil
- 5g (1 tsp) Mexican Spice Mix (pg. 69)
- 70g (½ medium) Red Onion
- 230g (2) Roma Tomatoes
- 60g (¼) Red Capsicum
- 2 stalks Spring Onion (green part only)
- 1 Baby Cos Lettuce

GUACAMOLE
- 1 large Avocado
- ¼ tsp fine Sea Salt
- ¼ tsp ground Black Pepper
- ½ tsp Mexican Spice Mix (pg. 69)
- Juice of ½ fresh Lime

SERVING
- Organic Corn Chips
- Fresh Coriander Leaves

Prep. Time: 15 min
Cook Time: 30 min
Serves: 4

DIRECTIONS – Traditional Only

Traditional ~ In a small saucepan, add the rinsed rice, vegetable stock paste, mexican spice mix and lime juice. Cover and bring to a boil then reduce the heat and simmer for 10 MIN or until the water is absorbed.

Peel the sweet potato. Cut the sweet potato, cauliflower and pineapple into 2cm pieces. Place onto a lined baking tray. Drizzle with olive oil and the mexican spice mix and toss to combine. Spread the mix out evenly on the tray. Bake in the oven at 180°C for 30 MIN.

Finely dice the red onion, tomatoes, capsicum and spring onion. Add these to a large bowl, stir together and set aside. When the roast vegetables are done, add them to this raw salad mix and toss together to combine.

Slice the lettuce finely and set aside.

Make your guacamole by mashing together the avocado, salt, pepper, lime juice and mexican spice mix.

~ ~ ~ ~ ~ ~ ~ ~ ~ ~ ~ ~ ~ ~ ~

Layer the ingredients in the following order:

1. Cover the bottom and sides of your serving bowl with some lettuce. Add a portion of the cooked rice on top and spread it out a little.
2. Add your vegetable + salad mix. Place some guacamole on top along with some corn chips.
3. Sprinkle with fresh coriander leaves.

DINNER

LENTIL LASAGNE

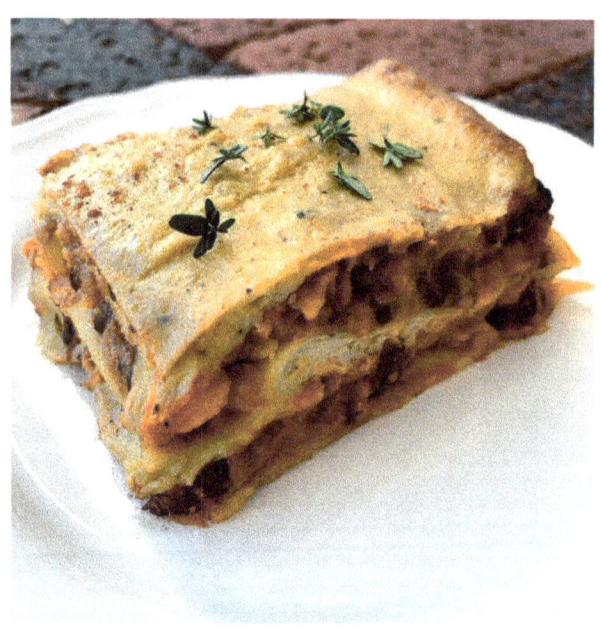

INGREDIENTS

- 1 packet Lasagne Sheets

FILLING

- 75g (½ medium) Brown Onion
- 3 Garlic Cloves
- 60g (1) Portobello Mushroom
- 140g (½) Zucchini
- 325g (½ large) Eggplant
- 125g (¼ medium) Sweet Potato
- 320g (¼) Butternut Pumpkin
- 15g (1 Tbsp) Olive Oil
- 1 x 700g jar Passata
- 40g (2 Tbsp) Vegetable Stock Paste (pg. 65)
- ½ tsp ground Black Pepper
- 1 tsp dried Oregano
- ¼ cup fresh Basil Leaves OR 1 tsp dried Basil
- 1 x 400g tinned Organic Black Lentils

BECHAMEL SAUCE

- 140g (1 cup) Unsalted Cashews
- 980g (1 L) Organic Soy Milk (this gives the best creaminess)
- 80g (½ cup) Plain Wholemeal Flour
- 30g (½ cup) Nutritional Yeast Flakes
- 10g (2 tsp) English Mustard
- 5g (2 tsp) Onion Powder
- 1 tsp Garlic Powder
- 1 tsp fine Sea Salt
- ½ tsp ground Black Pepper

SERVING

- Ground Paprika
- Fresh Thyme Leaves

DINNER

LENTIL LASAGNE (CONTINUED)

Prep. Time: 15 min
Cook Time: 55 min
Serves: 6

DIRECTIONS

1. Place the cashews into a heat proof bowl, cover the nuts with boiling water, place a lid on top and set aside for 10-15 MIN.
2. Drain off the excess liquid.

FILLING

Traditional ~ To make the filling, peel and finely dice the onion and garlic. Finely dice the mushroom. Peel the sweet potato. Cut the zucchini, eggplant and sweet potato into 1cm cubes. Place the onion, garlic, mushroom, zucchini, eggplant and sweet potato into a large frypan and add the olive oil. Cook on a medium heat for 10 MIN, stirring frequently.

Add the passata, vegetable stock paste, black pepper, oregano and basil leaves to the frypan. Stir together and cook for 5 MIN. Rinse and drain the tinned lentils, then add to the frypan and stir briefly (until they are mixed through).

Thermomix ~ To make the filling, peel the sweet potato and pumpkin. Roughly chop the mushroom, zucchini, eggplant, sweet potato and pumpkin. Add these along with the peeled onion and garlic into the TM bowl. Chop for 20 SEC / SP 4. Add the olive oil and cook for 8 MIN / VAROMA / REVERSE / SP 2.

Add the passata, vegetable stock paste, black pepper, oregano and basil into the TM bowl and cook for 5 MIN / 100°C / REVERSE / SP 2.

Rinse and drain the tinned lentils and add into the TM bowl. Mix for 10 SEC / REVERSE / SP 3. Place the filling into the Thermoserver. Rinse and dry the TM bowl.

BECHAMEL SAUCE

Traditional ~ To make the bechamel sauce you will need to add the drained cashews into a small saucepan along with the remaining bechamel sauce ingredients. Over a medium–low heat, stir and cook until the sauce thickens (approx. 10 MIN). Using a stick mixer, blend until the sauce becomes smooth.

Thermomix ~ To make the bechamel sauce, add the drained cashews into the TM bowl along with the remaining bechamel sauce ingredients. Cook for 7 MIN / 80°C / SP 4.

~ ~ ~ ~ ~ ~ ~ ~ ~ ~ ~ ~ ~ ~ ~

Using a lasagne dish, spread a couple tablespoons of the bechamel sauce onto the bottom of the dish. Then begin layering in the following order:

1. Lasagne sheets
2. Filling
3. Bechamel sauce

Repeat until your dish is full. Sprinkle a little paprika and thyme leaves over the top.

Bake in the oven at 180°C for 30-40 MIN.

NOTES

If served straight away, the structure of the sliced lasagne may not hold like a traditional lasagne, however it still tastes amazing.

It can be made ahead of time, then cooled so the bechamel sauce thickens – just reheat in the oven before serving on plates.

DINNER

MISO SOUP

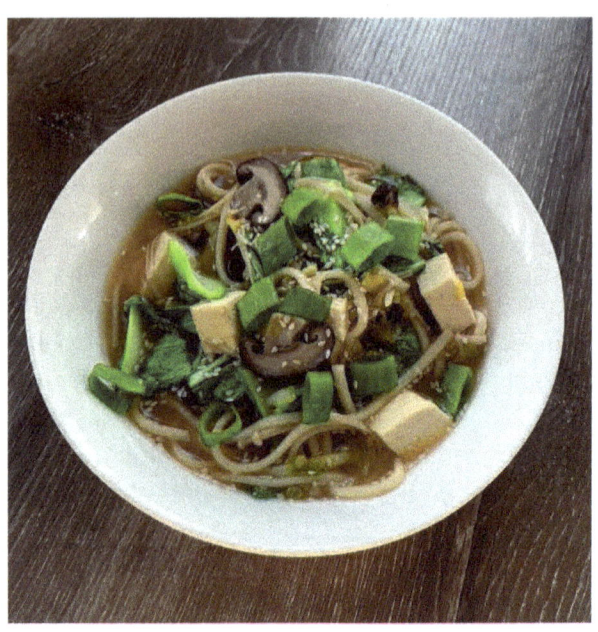

Prep. Time: 10 min
Cook Time: 15 min
Serves: 4

INGREDIENTS

- 4cm piece Fresh Ginger OR 3 tsp Ginger Powder
- 2 Garlic Cloves
- 15g (1 Tbsp) Organic Tamari Sauce
- 20g (1 Tbsp) Organic White Miso Paste
- ⅛ tsp Cayenne Pepper
- 5g (1 tsp) Vegetable Stock Paste (pg. 65)
- 980g (1L) Filtered Water
- 250g Organic Tofu
- 200g (½) Savoy Cabbage
- 100g (4 large) Shiitake Mushrooms
- 100g Oyster Mushrooms
- ¼ tsp Reishi Powder (optional)
- 140g Organic Udon Noodles
- 2 heads of Bok Choy (stalks + leaves)
- 10g (1 Tbsp) Sesame Seeds

SERVING

- 2 stalks Spring Onions (green part only)

DIRECTIONS

Traditional ~ Peel and finely dice the ginger and garlic. Place these into a large saucepan along with the tamari sauce, miso paste, cayenne pepper, vegetable stock paste and filtered water. Bring to a boil then reduce the heat to a simmer.

Thinly slice the shiitake and oyster mushrooms. Thinly slice the cabbage. Snap the noodles in half. Add these all into the saucepan with the reishi powder and cook over a low heat for 10 MIN, stirring occasionally.

Cut the tofu into 2cm cubes and roughly chop the bok choy. Add these into the saucepan along with the sesame seeds and stir gently for 2 MIN.

Thermomix ~ Peel the ginger and garlic and place into the TM bowl. Chop for 3 SEC / SP 7. Scrape down the sides of the bowl. Add the tamari sauce, miso paste, cayenne pepper, vegetable stock paste and filtered water. Cook for 5 MIN / 100°C / SP 1.

Thinly slice the shiitake and oyster mushrooms. Thinly slice the cabbage. Snap the noodles in half. Add these along with the reishi powder to the TM bowl. Cook for 8 MIN / 100°C / REVERSE / SP 2.

Roughly chop the bok choy. Cut the tofu into 2cm cubes. Add to the TM bowl along with the sesame seeds. Cook for 2 MIN / 100°C / REVERSE / SP STIR.

~ ~ ~ ~ ~ ~ ~ ~ ~ ~ ~ ~ ~ ~ ~

Serve in bowls and sprinkle sliced spring onions on top.

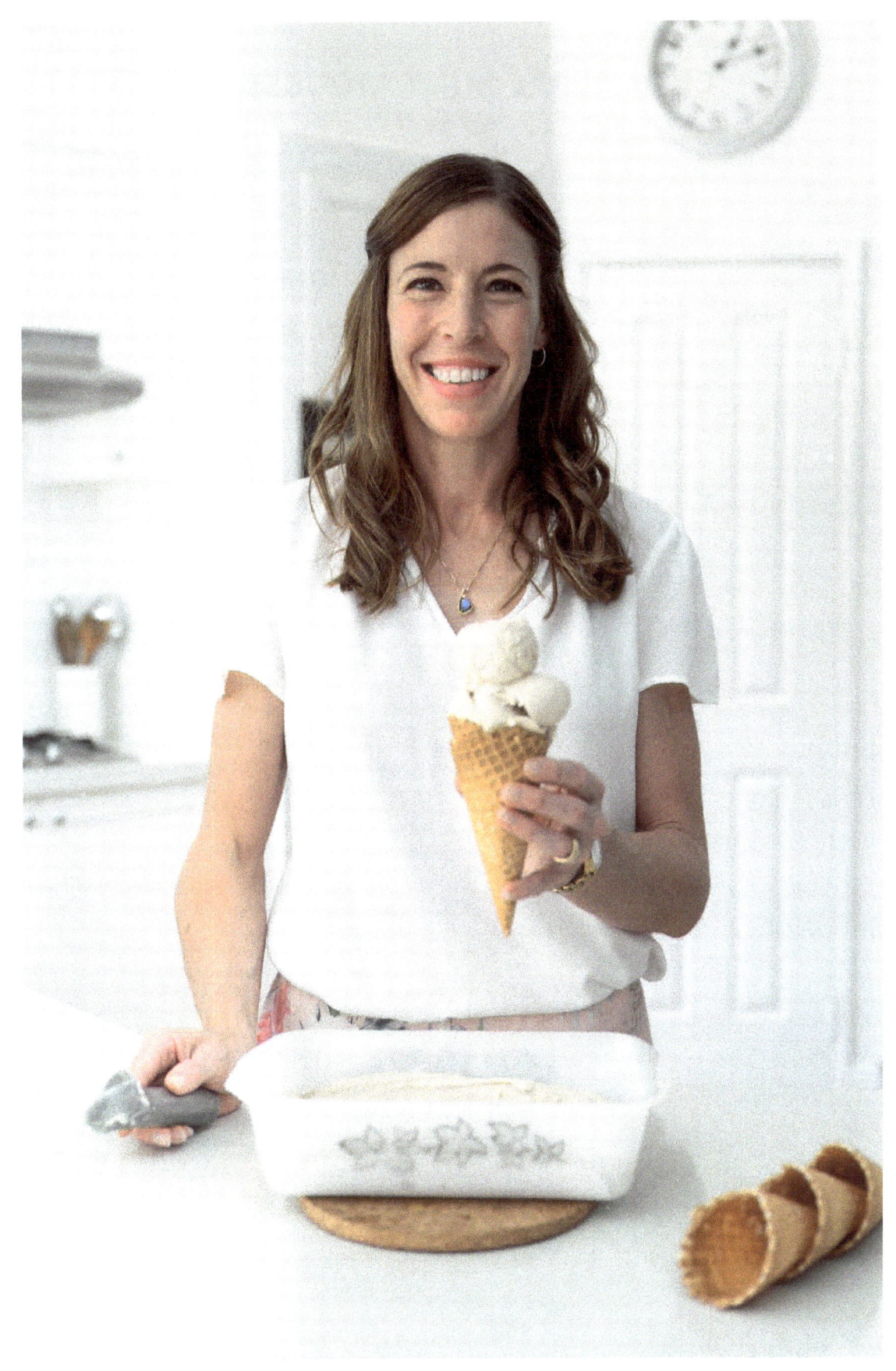

DESSERT

DESSERT

CHOCOLATE MINT MOUSSE

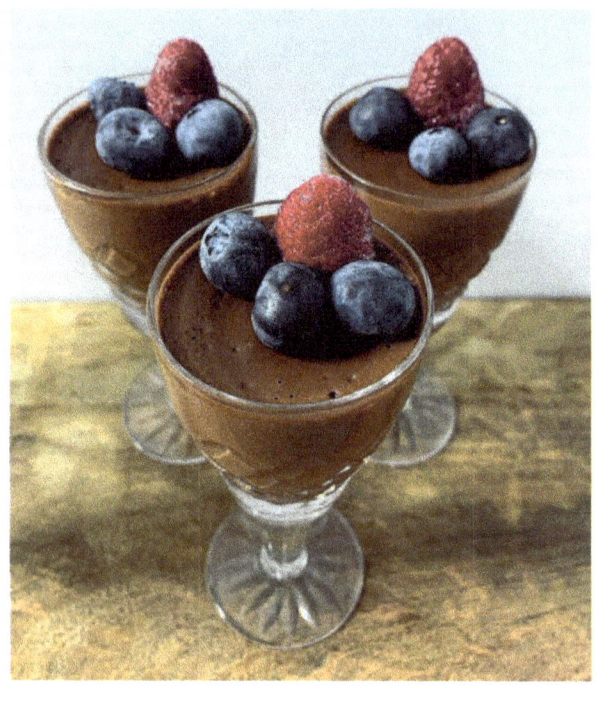

INGREDIENTS

- Liquid from 1 x 400g tinned Organic Chickpeas (also known as aquafaba)
- 160g Chocolate (dairy free + good quality)
- 2 drops Peppermint Essential Oil (food grade)

SERVING
- Fresh Berries

Prep. Time:	Make Time:	Serves:
5 min	7 min	5-6

DIRECTIONS

Traditional ~ Strain the liquid from the tinned chickpeas into a large sized bowl. Using an electric whisk, whisk until stiff peaks occur (this should take around 5 MIN).

Using the double boiler method, break the chocolate into small pieces. Add the chocolate pieces to a large glass bowl and set on top of a saucepan filled with enough water so it doesn't touch the glass bowl. Melt the chocolate over a low heat, stirring regularly.

Once the chocolate has melted, remove the bowl from the saucepan. Add a couple drops of peppermint essential oil and stir through. Then gently fold in the aquafaba. Keep folding until the chocolate and aquafaba are combined.

Thermomix ~ Insert the butterfly attachment into the TM bowl. Strain the liquid from the tinned chickpeas into the TM bowl. Whisk for 3 MIN / SP 4. Empty the fluffy aquafaba into a separate large bowl. Clean and dry the TM bowl.

Break the chocolate into pieces and add to the cleaned TM bowl. Grate for 8 SEC / SP 9. Melt for 3 MIN / 50°C / SP 2. Add the whisked aquafaba and peppermint essential oil into the melted chocolate. Mix for 10 SEC / REVERSE / SP 4.

~ ~ ~ ~ ~ ~ ~ ~ ~ ~ ~ ~ ~ ~ ~

Pour the mousse into sherry glasses and then place into the fridge for 40 MIN to set.

TO SERVE

Top with fresh berries and enjoy.

DESSERT

BERRY SORBET

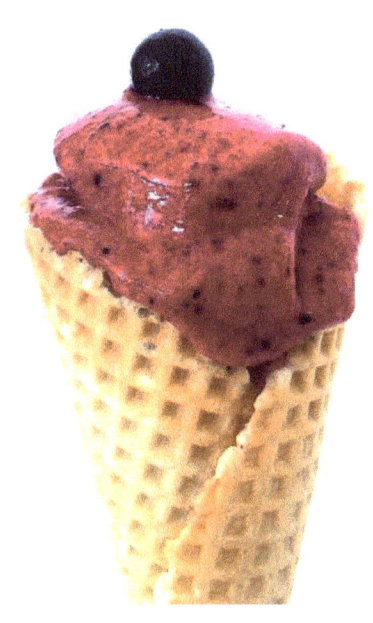

INGREDIENTS

- 60g (¼ cup) Organic Raw Sugar
- 170g (2 large) Bananas
- 100g (¾ cup) Organic Frozen Blueberries
- 250g (2 ½ cups) Organic Frozen Raspberries
- 10g (2 tsp) fresh Lemon Juice

SERVING
- Wafer Cones
- Frozen Berries

Prep. Time:	Cook Time:	Serves:
2 min	N/A	4

DIRECTIONS

Traditional ~ Cut the bananas into pieces and set aside. Add the raw sugar to a food processor and mill (alternatively, use ½ cup icing sugar). Add the remaining ingredients, including the bananas to the food processor and blend until combined.

Thermomix ~ Roughly cut the bananas into pieces and set aside. Add the raw sugar to the TM bowl and mill for 10 SEC / SP 10. Add the remaining ingredients, including the bananas and blend for 1 MIN / SP 5.

~ ~ ~ ~ ~ ~ ~ ~ ~ ~ ~ ~ ~ ~ ~

TO SERVE

Scoop the sorbet into wafer cones or bowls and top with any additional frozen berries.

NOTES

Serve immediately as it melts quickly.

DESSERT

PEANUT BUTTER CHOCOLATE

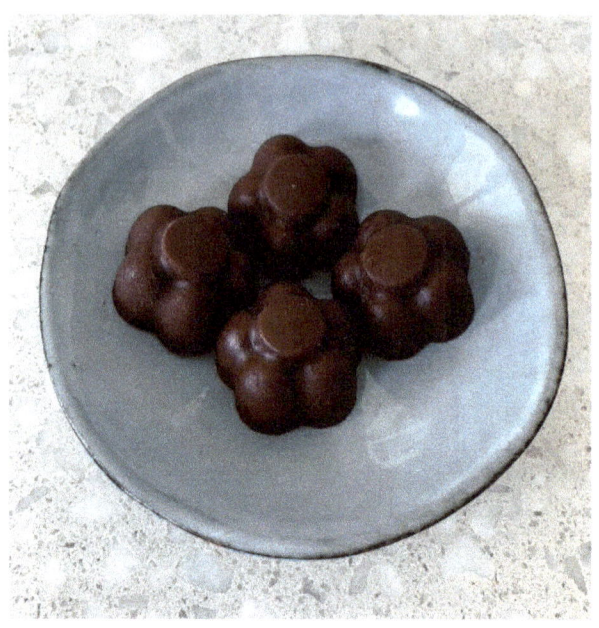

INGREDIENTS

- 200g (1 ⅔ cups) Cacao Butter Buttons
- 60g (¾ cup) Organic Cacao Powder
- 80g (4 Tbsp) Pure Maple Syrup
- 75g (¼ cup) Smooth Peanut Butter (good quality)
- ⅛ tsp fine Sea Salt

Prep. Time:	Cook Time:	Makes:
5 min	25 min	350g

DIRECTIONS

Traditional ~ In a small saucepan add the cacao butter buttons Melt on a low heat, stirring frequently for 10-15 MIN.

Add the remaining ingredients and continue to stir for another 10 MIN. Use a stick mixer to blend the chocolate into a smooth liquid consistency.

Thermomix ~ Add the cacao buttons to the TM bowl and melt for 15 MIN / 37°C / SP 2.

Add the remaining ingredients to the TM bowl and melt for 10 MIN / 37°C / SP 1. Blend for 10 SEC / SP 5.

~~~~~~~~~~~~~~~

Pour into silicone moulds and sprinkle each with a little extra fine sea salt. Place into the freezer to set for at least 1 HR.

NOTES

Store in an airtight container the fridge.

These will stay room temperature stable as well.

DESSERT

EASY RAW CHOCOLATE

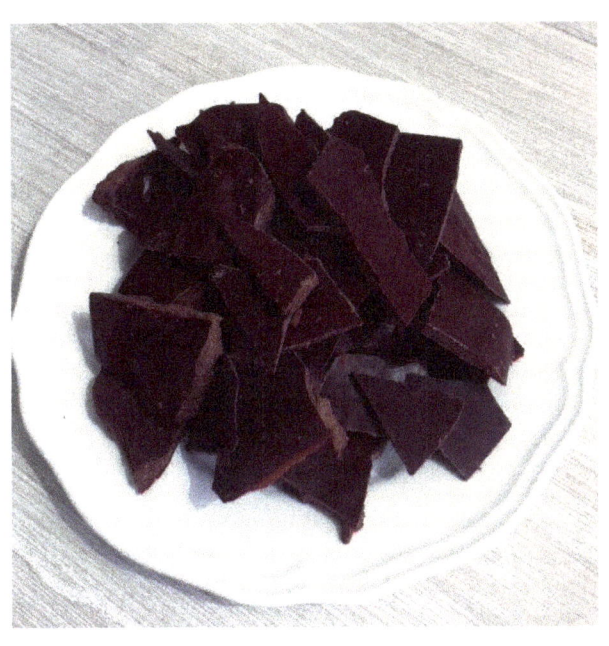

Prep. Time: 5 min
Cook Time: 5 min
Makes: 350g

DIRECTIONS

Traditional ~ Add the coconut butter and coconut oil to a saucepan and melt together over a low heat for 5 MIN. Once melted, remove the saucepan from the heat. Add the remaining ingredients and stir until combined.

Thermomix ~ Add the coconut butter and coconut oil into the TM bowl and melt together for 4 MIN / 37°C / SP STIR. Add the remaining ingredients and mix for 10 SEC / SP 3.

~ ~ ~ ~ ~ ~ ~ ~ ~ ~ ~ ~ ~ ~ ~

Line a baking tray with baking paper. Pour the chocolate mixture onto the lined tray.

Sprinkle one of the toppings (if desired) over the chocolate. Pecans are delicious along with orange food grade essential oil.

Place the tray into the freezer for 20 MIN to set. Once set, remove from the freezer and break into bite size pieces.

INGREDIENTS

- 100g (½ cup) Organic Coconut Butter
- 110g (½ cup) Organic Coconut Oil
- 60g (¾ cup) Organic Cacao Powder
- 60g (3 Tbsp) Pure Maple Syrup
- 8 drops Peppermint OR Wild Orange Essential Oil (food grade) - optional

TOPPINGS (optional)
- Pecans
- Freeze Dried Fruit (additive free)
- Frozen Blueberries

NOTES

Store in an airtight container in the freezer for up to 4 weeks (if not eaten before then).

DESSERT

APPLE CRUMBLE

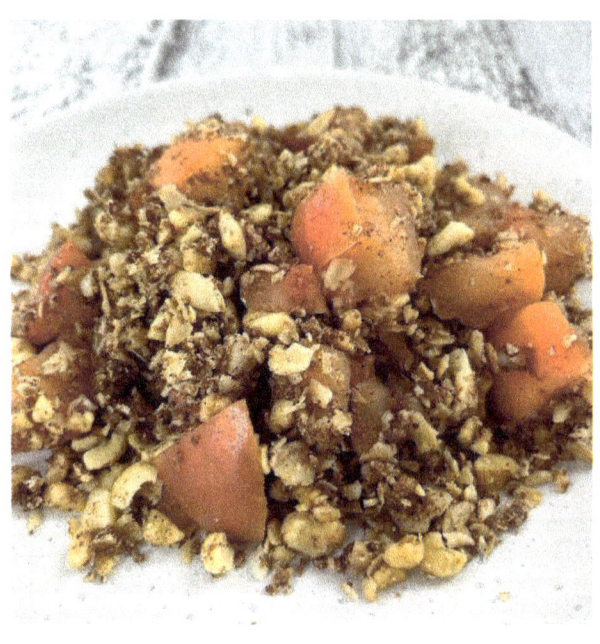

Prep. Time:	Cook Time:	Serves:
10 min	25 min	4

DIRECTIONS

Traditional ~ Roughly chop the nuts. Place the chopped nuts into a large bowl and add the remaining crumble ingredients. Stir until combined, then set aside.

Wash, core and cut the apples into 2cm pieces.

Add the apples, water and cinnamon to a medium saucepan and stir together. Cover and cook on a medium heat for 10 MIN. Once cooked, strain off the excess liquid.

Thermomix ~ Add all the crumble ingredients into the TM bowl and mix for 10 SEC / SP 4. Empty into a separate bowl and set aside. Clean and dry the TM bowl.

Wash, core and cut the apples into 2cm pieces.

Add the cubed apple pieces, water and cinnamon to the TM bowl and cook for 7 MIN / 80°C / SP 1. Once cooked, carefully strain off the excess liquid.

~ ~ ~ ~ ~ ~ ~ ~ ~ ~ ~ ~ ~ ~ ~

Add the stewed apple to a large baking dish and press gently to create an even layer. Top with the crumble mixture. Gently press the crumble mixture on top of the stewed apples.

Bake in the oven at 180°C for 15 MIN. Allow to cool slightly before serving.

NOTES

Store in an airtight container in the fridge for up to 2 days. Reheat any leftovers in the oven. For a gluten free option, use coconut flakes instead of rolled oats.

INGREDIENTS

CRUMBLE

- 80g (¾ cup) Walnuts
- 80g (½ cup) Unsalted Macadamia Nuts
- 80g (½ cup) Unsalted Cashews
- 80g (¾ cup) Organic Rolled Oats
- 30g (2 Tbsp) Organic Coconut Oil
- 30g (2 Tbsp) Brown Sugar
- 10g (1 Tbsp) Cinnamon

STEWED APPLE

- 660g (5) Large Red Apples
- 160g (⅔ cup) Filtered Water
- 1 tsp Cinnamon

DESSERT

SALTED CARAMEL ICE CREAM

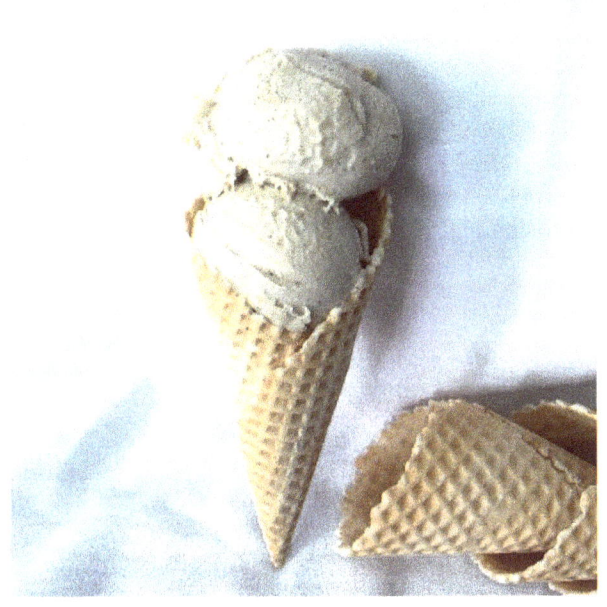

Prep. Time:	Cook / Freeze Time:	Makes:
10 min	18 min / 16 hrs	1 L

INGREDIENTS

- 200g (1 ½ cups) Unsalted Cashews
- 200g (1 cup) Organic Raw Sugar
- 30g (2 Tbsp) Organic Coconut Oil
- 80g (¼ cup) Pure Maple Syrup
- 10g (2 tsp) Organic Vanilla Bean Paste
- 5g (1 tsp) fine Sea Salt
- 1 x 400ml tinned Organic Coconut Cream

SERVING
- Wafer Cones

DIRECTIONS

1. Place the cashews into a glass heat proof dish. Cover with boiling water. Set aside for 1 hour. Drain and discard the liquid.

Traditional ~ Add the sugar, coconut oil, maple syrup, vanilla paste, salt and coconut cream to a saucepan and stir over a medium heat for 5 MIN. Set aside and allow to cool.

Place the drained cashews into a large bowl with the cooled liquid mixture. Using beaters, blend until you have a smooth consistency. Pour the ice cream into a metal loaf tin. Place in the freezer for 3-4 HRS to partially freeze.

Once partially frozen, tip the ice cream into a large bowl. Beat for 1 MIN. Pour the ice cream back into the metal tin and place into the freezer for 12 HRS to set.

Thermomix ~ Add the sugar, coconut oil, maple syrup, vanilla paste, salt and coconut cream to the TM bowl. Mix for 5 SEC / SP 5. Scrape down the sides of the TM bowl. Cook for 5 MIN / VAROMA / SP 1. Let this sit until the cashews are ready.

Add the drained cashews to the TM bowl. Blend for 1 MIN / SP 7 - gradually working up to SP 9. Pour the ice cream into a metal loaf tin. Place in the freezer for 3-4 HRS to partially freeze.

Once partially frozen, tip the ice cream into the TM bowl and mix for 1 MIN / SP 5. Pour the ice cream back into the metal tin and place in the freezer for 12 HRS to set.

~ ~ ~ ~ ~ ~ ~ ~ ~ ~ ~ ~ ~ ~ ~

TO SERVE

Scoop into wafer cones or bowls. Store in an airtight container in the freezer for up to 4 weeks.

DESSERT

CHEWY CHOC CARAMEL FUDGE

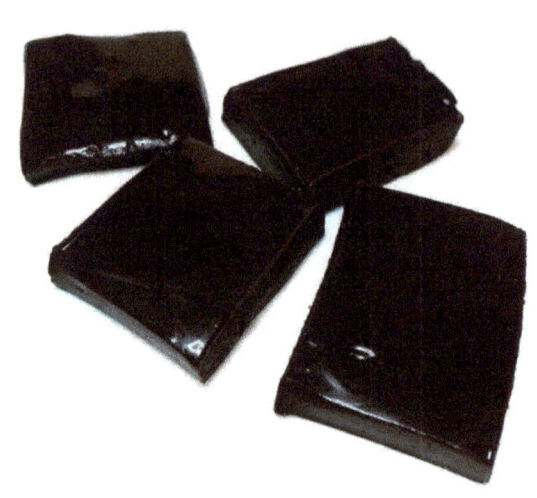

Prep. Time:	Cook Time:	Makes:
5 min	6 min	250g

DIRECTIONS

Traditional ~ Add all the ingredients into a small saucepan. Melt together over a medium–low heat, stirring regularly for 6 MIN.

Thermomix ~ Add all the ingredients into the TM bowl. Cook for 6 MIN / 70°C / SP 1.

~~~~~~~~~~~~~~~~

Line a small square tin with baking paper and pour the mixture in. Place in the freezer to set for 1 HR.

Remove from the tin and cut the fudge into bite size pieces.

INGREDIENTS

- 200g (½ cup) Organic Rice Malt Syrup
- 45g (3 Tbsp) Organic Coconut Oil
- 60g (¾ cup) Organic Cacao Powder
- 5g (1 tsp) Organic Vanilla Bean Paste
- Pinch of fine Sea Salt

NOTES

The fudge should be glossy.

Work quickly before your warm hands start to melt it.

Store in an airtight container in the fridge for up to 1 week.

DESSERT

PEPPERMINT ICE

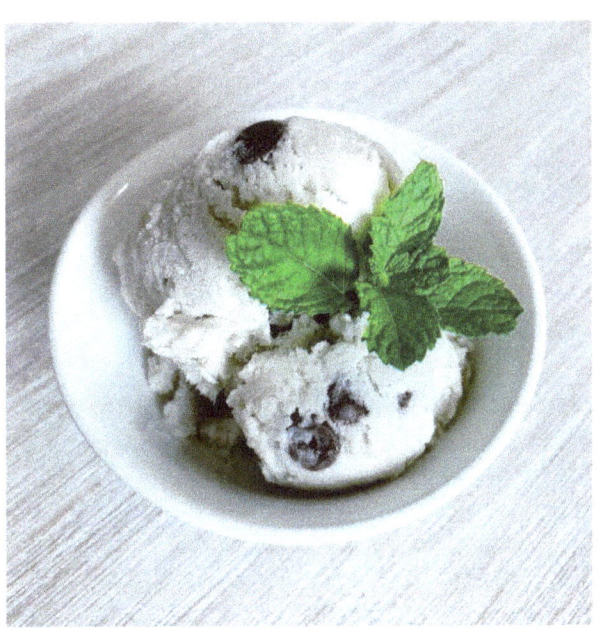

Prep. Time:	Cook / Freeze Time:	Makes:
5 min	7 min / 16 hr	1.5 L

DIRECTIONS

Traditional ~ Add the coconut cream, coconut milk, sugar and maple syrup into a saucepan. Cook for 5 MIN stirring regularly over a medium–low heat.

Pour into a 1.5L glass heat proof dish and place into the freezer for 4 HRS until partially frozen.

Remove from the freezer, pour the contents into a large mixing bowl. Using beaters on a medium speed, beat for 2 MIN until smooth and glossy.

Add the peppermint essential oil and chocolate chips (if using) and stir gently to combine.

Thermomix ~ Add the coconut cream, coconut milk, sugar and maple syrup into the TM bowl. Mix for 5 SEC / SP 5. Then cook for 5 MIN / VAROMA / SP 1.

Pour into a 1.5L glass heat proof dish and place into the freezer for 4 HRS until partially frozen.

Remove from the freezer, pour the contents back into the clean TM bowl, insert the butterfly attachment and whisk for 2 MIN / SP 3.

Remove the butterfly attachment, add the peppermint oil and chocolate chips (if using), and mix for 1 MIN / REVERSE / SP 3.

~ ~ ~ ~ ~ ~ ~ ~ ~ ~ ~ ~ ~ ~

Pour the contents back into the glass dish and place in the freezer to set overnight if possible.

TO SERVE

Scoop into wafer cones or bowls. Store in an airtight container in the freezer for up to 4 weeks.

INGREDIENTS

- 1 x 400ml tinned Organic Coconut Cream
- 1 x 400ml tinned Organic Coconut Milk
- 110g (½ cup) Organic Raw Sugar
- 80g (¼ cup) Pure Maple Syrup
- 10-12 drops Peppermint Essential Oil (food grade)
- 100g (½ cup) Chocolate Chips – dairy free (optional)

SERVING

- Wafer Cones (optional)

NOTES

The consistency of this may depend on the brand of coconut cream and coconut milk that's used. Use a fork to scrape the mixture into ice.

DESSERT

FUDGE CHOC POPS

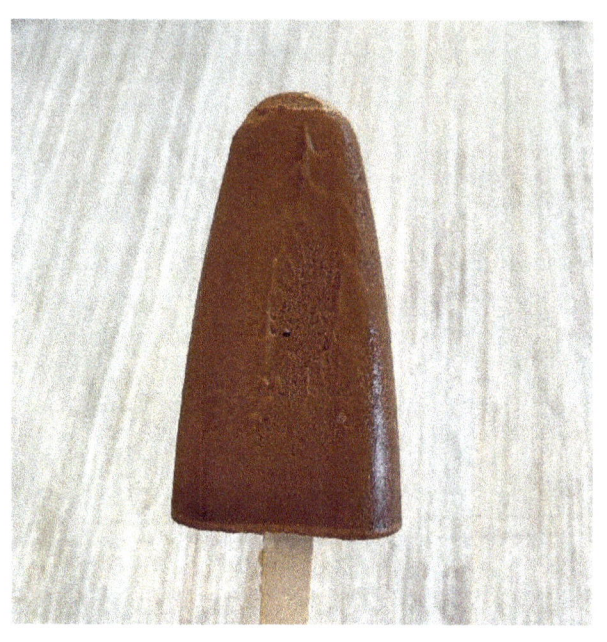

INGREDIENTS

- 1 x 400ml tinned Organic Coconut Cream
- 1 x 400ml tinned Organic Coconut Milk
- 85g (1 cup) Organic Cacao Powder
- 215g (⅔ cup) Pure Maple Syrup
- 10g (2 tsp) Organic Vanilla Bean Paste
- Pinch of fine Sea Salt

Prep. Time:	Cook / Freeze Time:	Makes:
5 min	1 min / 4 hrs	16

DIRECTIONS

Traditional ~ Add all the ingredients into a large bowl. Using beaters, beat together for 1 MIN or until the mixture is smooth.

Thermomix ~ Add all ingredients into the TM bowl and mix for 15 SEC / SP 8. Make sure the mixture is smooth before pouring.

~ ~ ~ ~ ~ ~ ~ ~ ~ ~ ~ ~ ~ ~ ~

Pour into popsicle moulds and place into the freezer for 4 HRS to set.

If using pop sticks, add once partially frozen and return to the freezer to set.

NOTES

These can be stored in the freezer for up to 1 week.

These are great for the kids too, especially on hot summer days.

www.ingramcontent.com/pod-product-compliance
Lightning Source LLC
Chambersburg PA
CBHW061536010526
44107CB00066B/2882